OPERATING THEATRE NURSING

Mary C Warren, SRN, RCNT

formerly Clinical Tutor, JBCNS
Course in Operating Theatre Nursing
Charing Cross Hospital, London

Harper & Row, Publishers
London

Cambridge
Hagerstown
Philadelphia
New York

San Francisco
Mexico City
Sao Paulo
Sydney

First published 1983

Harper and Row Ltd
28 Tavistock Street
London WC2E 7PN

British Library Cataloguing in Publication Data

Warren, Mary
  Operating theatre nursing.
  1. Operating room nursing
  I. Title
  610.73′677   RD32.3
  ISBN 0-06-318240-8

Typeset by Bookens, Saffron Walden, Essex
Printed and bound in Great Britain, by Butler & Tanner, Frome and London.

CONTENTS

FOREWORD

The aim in writing this book is to emphasise the importance of individual patient care in operating theatre nursing and to encourage a systematic and logical approach to the performance of practical procedures.

The chapter headings are related to the objectives contained in the outline curriculum for the Joint Board of Clinical Nursing Studies Course 176 and the text is intended to provide basic information that will be complemented by the specialist knowledge that is imparted by experienced nurses in the clinical situation.

It is hoped that the material in the book will be of general interest to operating theatre staff and will help to meet the needs of teachers and learners in operating theatres. Although operating theatre nursing is practised by male as well as female nurses and operating department assistants, for convenience, the nurse is referred to as 'she' and the patient as 'he' throughout the book.

CHAPTER 1

AN INTRODUCTION TO OPERATING THEATRE NURSING

Objectives

The nurse will be able to:

1 Relate the history and development of operating theatre nursing.
2 Describe the role of the nurse in the operating theatre.
3 Name the stages of the nursing process.
4 Enumerate the fundamental elements of effective communication.

The development of operating theatre nursing

Although there is no recorded date for the introduction of operating theatre nursing as a speciality, it was probably at the end of the nineteenth century that it all began. Until that time the nurse had prepared the patient for surgery, handed swabs and sutures during the operation and cared for him during the postoperative period. As the surgery was carried out on the bed, or a spare table in the ward, this seemed a satisfactory arrangement. Improvements in asepsis and anaesthetic techniques led to great advances in surgery and an increase in the number of operations undertaken. Hospitals built special departments called operating theatres, where surgery was performed by experienced surgeons and watched by medical students.

The surgeons depended on the nurses for the preparation of instruments and sutures, the cleaning and maintenance of equipment and assistance at operations. The nurses were proud of their role as handmaiden and assistant to the surgeon and worked diligently to provide the best possible conditions for surgery and to develop skills in handling instruments and equipment. The theatre nurse became a specialist working within the operating theatre while the surgical ward nurse assumed responsibility for the preoperative preparation and postoperative care of the patient.

In each hospital the operating department was controlled by the sister in charge whose responsibilities included the organisation and management of the theatres, the ordering of stock and equipment and assisting as scrub nurse at operations. The work was arduous and demanding and the nurses worked long hours, so it is not surprising that theatre staff found few opportunities for meeting and exchanging ideas with other nurses involved in the same speciality.

The Second World War brought changes in the operating theatre as in many other spheres. The technicians and auxilliary staff did valuable work in assisting in the preparation and sterilising of equipment and became permanent members of the theatre team. Meanwhile, the theatre nurses' knowledge was extended to include an appreciation of the techniques of surgery and anaesthesia and an understanding of the intricacies of the new and sophisticated equipment. More recently, operating theatre nurses have accepted the responsibility of caring for patients in the recovery room during the postanaesthesia period and it is becoming generally recognised that this involvement should be further extended if the individually planned care that is instituted on the ward is to be continued while the patient is in the operating department. Nurses who are able to visit patients before operations can identify the potential problems and plan for the patient's comfort and safety during his operation. Fears and anxieties can be dispelled during a preoperative interview and the patient is often reassured by talking with the nurse who will be present at his operation. These visits also offer valuable opportunities for establishing good relationships and cooperation between ward and theatre staff.

The present day theatre nurse faces fresh challenges with the advances in transplant and reconstructive surgery which offer exciting possibilities for prolonging life and demand a wide knowledge of the new techniques and materials involved.

The role of the nurse in the operating theatre

The nurse's role in the operating theatre is to provide nursing care and safety for the patient, from the time of his arrival in the department until his return to the ward after surgery.

Knowledge and experience are requisites for working in such a specialised area. The nurse becomes a member of a skilled team which includes doctors, nurses, operating department assistants, and ancillary staff, all of whom are specialists working together to achieve the best results for the patient.

The qualities of diligence and conscientiousness which are developed during the basic nurse training are especially important in operating theatre nursing when the patient is totally dependent on other people to act for him while he is unconscious.

Manual dexterity is required, to cope with technical skills and the management of equipment, but an empathy with the patient and an ability to anticipate and provide for his physical and emotional well being is of equal importance.

The theatre nurse's job is often demanding but the close team work generates a sense of involvement which enthuses theatre nurses and encourages them to strive continually to improve standards of care and to master new techniques.

The responsibilities of staff in the operating theatre

1 The provision of a safe environment in which surgery can be performed.
2 The provision of total patient care during the perioperative period (which includes pre-, intra-, and postoperative phases).
3 Acting as advocate for the patient to guard his safety and his dignity during periods of sedation and unconsciousness.

The duties of nurses in the operating department

1 Preoperative care
  The reception nurse identifies the patient and is responsible for providing safety and comfort in the transfer area.
  The anaesthetic nurse assists the anaesthetist and cares for the patient during the induction of anaesthesia.
2 Intraoperative care
  The scrub nurse in the operating theatre assists the surgeon and maintains a sterile field.
  The circulating nurse anticipates and supplies the needs of the scrubbed team during the operation.

3 Postoperative care
   The recovery nurse records observations and continues to give
   nursing care until the patient is able to return to the ward.

The nursing process

The nursing process represents an intellectual approach to individual
patient care which is being developed in all branches of nursing. The
problem-solving and systematic approach involves assessing the patients
needs and identifying potential problems, planning the care to be given,
implementing the proposed plans and evaluating the outcome and the
effect on the patient.

The stages of the nursing process

1 Assessment
   The assessment of the individual patient's needs and the identification
   of potential problems is achieved by:
     a Observation of the patient.
     b Utilisation of data from the medical and nursing histories.
     c Conversation with the patient during a preoperative inter-
        view.
2 Planning
     a Realistic goals for the patient to achieve, are established.
     b Plans are made for appropriate action to provide safety and
        comfort for the patient.
     c The plans are recorded and communicated to all the personnel
        involved in the implementation.
3 Implementation
     a The planned actions are implemented or, if necessary, revised.
     b The nursing actions are recorded.
4 Evaluation
   The results of nursing care are appraised and evaluated to determine
   whether the preset goals were achieved.

In countries where the nursing process is used to provide planned
individual patient care in the operating theatre, many nurses are
convinced that the quality of care has been enhanced. They are
enthusiastic in expressing confidence in the value of preoperative and
postoperative visiting to alleviate stress and anxiety.

Communication

The communication of relevant information and data is an essential factor in theatre nursing and in the successful use of the nursing process. Forethought and logical thinking are the first requirements in developing an expertise in communication with patients, members of the surgical team and the ward staff.

Guidelines for establishing good communication

1 Use simple words and state times and places precisely.
2 Make sure that one instruction has been understood before proceeding to the next subject. Misunderstanding can arise from hearing defects, language difficulties and anxiety.
3 Be specific and address communications directly to the person concerned.
4 Listen to the other person's point of view.
5 Record events in writing.
6 Complete documents promptly and accurately.

The safety of the patient and the efficient organisation of the theatre depends on the establishment of good communications between all the members of the operating room staff.

Communications with patients

Preoperative interviews

A genuine interest in the patient as an individual, readiness to listen to him and an empathy with him in his present circumstances, are the first essentials for successful interviews with patients, prior to surgery.

Before embarking on a preoperative visit the nurse needs to gather as much information as possible about the patient. Perusal of the medical and nursing histories will provide the personal details that are required for documentary purposes and the ward nurse can often supply additional information from her observations and contact with the patient since his admission to the ward.

Having completed these preliminary investigations, the theatre nurse can approach the patient, greeting him by name and introducing herself while she explains the purpose of her visit. When she has established that the time is not inconvenient and the patient is able to talk to her, the nurse should seat herself beside him, where he can see her face.

During conversation, brief notes can be recorded on a form listing the data and observations that are needed in order to prepare a plan for the nursing care throughout the perioperative period. While he is talking the nurse may observe that the patient is uneasy and fidgeting nervously or showing other signs of hitherto unnoticed emotional stress.

During further conversation the cause of the anxiety may be revealed, offering the theatre nurse an opportunity to discuss the problem and to help allay anxiety and relieve tension. She will be able to answer questions about the preparations for surgery and explain the reasons for the procedures at the reception area of the operating department but when queries arise that cannot be satisfactorily answered by the theatre nurse, these problems must be communicated to an experienced person who is qualified and able to deal with the question.

Encouragement to practise suitable breathing exercises and muscle relaxation is often welcomed by the patient who appreciates an opportunity to contribute to his own treatment.

Having established a relationship with the patient the nurse is able to reassure him that the nurses in the operating department will be aware of his problems and prepared to support him throughout the time that he is in the theatre until his safe return to the ward.

Further reading

Gruendemann, B J (1977) The Surgical Patient. Behavioural Concepts for the Operating Room Nurse, Mosby

Hunt, M and Marks-Maran, D J (1981) Nursing Care Plans, HM&M

MacFarlane, J and Casteldine, G (1982) A Guide to the Practice of Nursing Using the Nursing Process, Mosby

Smith, V and Bass, T (1982) Communication for the Health Care Team, Harper & Row

CHAPTER 2

THE OPERATING THEATRE ENVIRONMENT

Objectives

The nurse will be able to:

1 Describe the function of the main areas of the operating department.
2 List the essential facilities and services in a modern operating department.
3 Outline possible routes for the movement of patients, staff and supplies within the department.
4 Describe the ventilation, air conditioning and air flow systems in the operating theatre.

The operating theatre environment

The first operating theatres were usually built as single units or as a twin unit with two operating theatres of identical design. These theatres provided adequate facilities for surgery in those hospitals which were established to serve the needs of local communities or to be centres for specialisation in one particular branch of surgery. Since the Second World War the policy has been to build large district hospitals with operating departments comprised of a number of theatres, grouped together, in order to make the best use of the Centralised Supply Services that have been developed.

Theatre design

Operating departments are self-contained units which often occupy an entire wing or floor of the hospital (Figure 2.1).

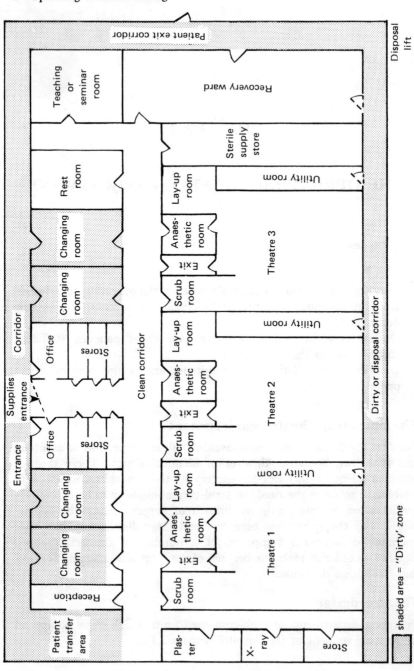

Figure 2.1   Plan of operating department.

Layout

The rooms of the department are arranged within a complex which is divided into 'clean' and 'dirty' zones:

1 An approach corridor from which the patients enter the transfer area and the staff enter the changing rooms.
2 A central or clean area or corridor giving access to theatre suites and supply rooms.
3 The exit or dirty area where used items are deposited ready for cleaning or disposal.

Areas of the operating department

The reception and transfer area

Patients are received into the department and their identity is checked when they are transferred from the ward bed or trolley to the theatre trolley before entering the clean zone.

Sterilising and supply areas

A Theatre Sterile Supply Unit (TSSU) where instruments and equipment are prepared and sterilised, may be situated in the clean zone and there is a storage place for presterilised packages that are delivered from a Central Sterile Supply Department (CSSD).

The operating suite

1 The anaesthetic room used for the induction of anaesthesia.
2 Operating theatre equipped with operating table and equipment.
3 Lay-up area for the preparation of sterile trolleys.
4 Scrub-up area for hand washing, gowning and gloving of the surgical team.
5 Utility room for the disposal and cleaning of used instruments and equipment.
6 Patient exit room, or space, provided with oxygen and suction for immediate postoperative care.

Recovery room

A room is prepared for the accommodation of patients on theatre trolleys or beds and is equipped with individual suction apparatus, oxygen supply and monitors for the observation and nursing of patients postoperatively, until they are able to return to the ward.

Storage rooms
Cupboards are needed for storage of equipment, laundry, medicines and domestic supplies.

Radiography facilities
Developing rooms and spaces are designated for the storage of X-ray machines, lead-lined aprons and films.

Staff changing rooms
Several rooms are reserved to provide space and privacy for personnel to change from outdoor clothing and uniform into clean theatre garments before entering the clean zone. These rooms are furnished with lockers for the safe storage of personal belongings and with shelving for a supply of theatre clothing. Toilet facilities and showers are installed in each changing room.

Rest rooms
Rest rooms with comfortable seating and facilities for the preparation of light refreshment, are used by the staff for relaxation during long spells of duty.

Teaching rooms
Conference or teaching rooms are an essential amenity in modern operating theatres. These rooms are used for in-service training and teaching, and for staff meetings.

Office accommodation
Office space is needed to accommodate medical and nursing secretarial staff and for the use of nursing administrators.

Communication control centre
An information desk and telephone switchboard are installed for the coordination and relaying of information to all areas of the theatre department.

Maintenance and repair facilities
Access panels and routes are used by the engineers to reach pipes, conduits and machines.

The fabric of the operating theatre

Colour
Soft colours that are restful and soothing for patients and staff are used in the main areas, with contrast colours to denote entrances and exits and to define 'clean' and 'dirty' zones.

Durability
Smooth scratch-proof surfaces, that are easily cleaned, will discourage dust from settling and bacterial growth from forming. Strong flooring is laid to withstand the damage caused by the movement of heavy equipment.

Safety
Antistatic rubber wheels fitted to metal trolleys and earthed conductive metal strips embedded in the flooring prevent the accumulation of static electricity in the operating theatre.

Cleaning
All furniture should be mobile and the surfaces uncluttered, to allow efficient cleaning with disinfectant agents.

Noise
To combat the persistent and jarring noises that cause stress and irritation to the staff and the patients, quiet flooring and swing doors are installed wherever possible and polypropylene bowls and dishes may be used in preference to stainless steel.

Traffic routes in the operating department

When a policy has been agreed that defines the utilisation of the theatres and the estimated number and type of operations to be performed, the routes or pathways are established for the movement of patients, staff and supplies. These routes follow a general direction which progresses from the clean to the dirty zones to minimise the risk of cross-infection if clean and unused items should come into contact with used equipment.

The route for patients

1 Patients arrive at the reception area.
2 Proceed to the holding area or the anaesthetic room.

3   Enter the operating theatre.
4   Transfer to the exit room or bay at the end of the operation.
5   Enter the recovery room.
6   Return to the surgical ward.

Staff routes

1   Enter the changing rooms.
2   Emerge into the clean zone wearing theatre clothing.
3   Enter the scrub-up area and the operating theatre.
4   Leave the theatre at the end of the operation by the patient exit door or the utility room.

Routes for supplies

1   Delivery of sterile and clean supplies at a special goods entrance.
2   Storage in the clean zone of the theatres.
3   Transfer to the utility room after use and removal by a separate disposal route.

Access facilities

1   Stairways provide access to the department for visitors and staff.
2   A lift is reserved for the transport of patients.
3   Separate routes are designated for the delivery of supplies and for the disposal of waste.

Ventilation and air conditioning

Controlled mechanical ventilation is installed to create a safe and comfortable environment for the patients and for the staff.

Ventilation methods

1   Outside air is drawn into ducts and passed through high resistance filters to remove dust particles.
2   This clean air is diffused through vents in the ceiling, creating a positive pressure within the theatre and forcing contaminated air to be discharged through wall outlets at floor level.
3   Heating and cooling systems are incorporated to maintain optimum conditions for comfort and safety at a temperature of 22°C and relative humidity approximately 55–60%.

4 The rate of air flow is regulated to give 16–20 changes of air per hour in the theatre.
5 Exhaled anaesthetic gases are channelled from the patient to the outside atmosphere by scavenging systems in the theatres, anaesthetic rooms and recovery rooms.

Hazards to efficient ventilation and air conditioning

1 The movement of personnel creates turbulence and deflection of the air flow.
2 Frequent opening and closing of doors causes variations in the pressure and the volume of air in the theatre.
3 Raised humidity levels create a risk of an accumulation of static electricity.
4 Dusty inlet grilles increase the amount of bacteria in the theatre atmosphere.
5 Outlet ducts which become blocked prevent the efficient extraction of contaminated air.
6 Filter screens that are not regularly maintained and renewed, decrease the efficiency of the system.

Laminar air flow systems

Ventilation units have been developed for use during surgery where there is a high risk of postoperative infection. Clean air is forced to flow in one direction at high velocity, in an effort to achieve a more effective elimination of bacteria from the theatre atmosphere. It is claimed that the speed at which the air flows prevents bacteria from settling around the wound area.

Vertical downward laminar flow systems

Sterile air flows from a diffuser plant over the operating table and in a downwards and outward direction at a controlled velocity of 60 feet per minute. The surgical team work in a clean air zone which may be enclosed by side panels or screens hung from the ceiling fitments. Recent designs have been produced that do not require full length floor-to-ceiling panels and are therefore less inhibiting and allow greater mobility of the scrub team.

Horizontal air flow

Specially designed units are built to deliver sterile air from a plant built into the wall of the operating theatre. The air is directed to flow horizontally over the operating table at high velocity, and out of the operating enclosure at ground level. This system necessitates using side curtains but allows the standard operating light to be used.

Total body exhaust systems

The wearer is enveloped in a floor length sterile gown and head covering with a length of flexible corrugated tubing attached to the inner side of the garment. Exhaled breath and contaminated, bacteria-laden air, which is emitted from the wearers body, is discharged through the corrugated tubing to a suction unit outside the operating table area.

Anaesthetic gas pollution

In the early 1970s attention was drawn to the dangers of waste anaesthetic gases in the operating theatre atmosphere and it was suggested that the inhalation of nitrous oxide and halothane could be the cause of the higher incidence of abortions and malformed babies amongst female anaesthetists. Research has not produced conclusive evidence that these or other waste gases are responsible for birth defects or for some of the physiological problems experienced by operating theatre staff, but the Department of Health and Social Security (DHSS 1976) circulated advice and recommendations on the installation of scavenging systems to remove exhaled gases from the theatres, the anaesthetic rooms and the recovery rooms.

Passive scavenging

A specially-fitted expiratory valve is incorporated in the anaesthetic circuit and the exhaled gases are channelled through tubing to a point in the ventilation system where it can safely be discharged to the outside air.

Active scavenging

Suction pumps or fans are used to draw the exhaled air from the room into the ducts, to be vented into the outer atmosphere. The scavenging unit can be a stable wall fitting or a mobile attachment suspended from a boom or a pendant. Activated charcoal is effective in reducing the levels of halothane, and of some other gases in the atmosphere. Cannisters containing this substance can be incorporated in anaesthetic circuits and air filter systems.

Lighting

Natural daylight is soft and pleasant to work in and does not induce the claustrophobic tendencies that are sometimes experienced by staff working in operating theatres which have been built without windows.

Operating theatre windows—requirements

1 Large enough to allow the maximum amount of daylight to enter.
2 Double glazed to eliminate disturbing noises.
3 Positioned and screened to ensure privacy and to prevent overlooking of the operating theatre.
4 Equipped with effective blinds or blacking-out devices for use when a darkened room is required.

Artificial light gives a constant light of even intensity. The absence of windows eliminates the problems of screening and darkening rooms.

Requirements for operating lights

1 Operating lights must be shadowless and easily manoeuvred.
2 An emergency lighting system must be available for use in the case of failure of the main supply.
3 Fluorescent lighting provides an efficient system for use in corridors, anaesthetic rooms and recovery rooms.

Oxygen and nitrous oxide gas supply

These gases are either supplied in cylinders or piped from a central manifold storage room and carried to wall or pendant outlets in the theatres and recovery rooms.

Communication systems

Telephone

Telephones are strategically sited to provide communication between personnel in all areas of the department and the central switchboard.

Intercommunication systems

Internal intercommunication devices relieve delays caused by the overloading of telephone lines and provide a quick and direct contact between members of the staff within the operating theatres.

Information desk

A central point from which the general theatre activity can be directed, messages relayed and patients and staff located.

Emergency systems

Warning and alarm signals are installed throughout the department for use in emergency situations only.

Further reading

Codes of Practice: The National Association of Theatre Nurses (22 Mount Parade, Harrogate, Yorks)

Howorth, F H (1981) What's in the Air in the Operating Theatre, NATNews, 18: 17–19

Reference

DHSS (1976) Health Services Development. Pollution of Operating Departments, etc, by Anaesthetic Gases, HC (76) 38

CHAPTER 3

PSYCHOLOGICAL ASPECTS OF OPERATING THEATRE NURSING

Objectives

The nurse will be able to:

1 Identify the causes of tension and stress in surgical patients.
2 Relate the causes of stress amongst members of the surgical team.
3 Discuss the importance of the team concept in operating theatre work.

The psychological problems of surgical patients

Modern techniques and elaborate equipment have increased the scope of surgery and reduced the risks of anaesthesia, but the emotional effects of surgical intervention can still present problems and hinder the recovery of the patient.

Causes of emotional stress

Apprehension

The patient who is admitted one or two days before an operation becomes accustomed to the surroundings and feels secure within the confines of the ward. He is increasingly apprehensive about leaving this environment for the unfamiliar world of the operating department peopled by staff who are strangers to him. The theatre nurse can inspire confidence by meeting the patient and reassuring him that the staff in the operating theatre are aware of his problems and will care for him while he is unconscious.

Fear

Fear is an emotion experienced to some degree by most patients before an operation and expressed in divers ways. A forced joviality may mask all kinds of fears and the apparently morose patient who replies in monosyllables may simply be afraid. Shocked patients who have been involved in an accident are frequently unable to utter a single word. The experienced nurse recognises these signs of fear and, with the help of the nursing history, can detect behavioural changes and respond to the patients need for reassurance by establishing eye contact, placing a reassuring hand on the patient's arm and attending to his bodily comfort quietly and effectively.

Disfigurement

The degree of disfigurement or mutilation that will result from the operation is a matter of deep concern to the patient. He may be convinced of the need for surgery and longing for relief of pain but the alteration to body image, and the effect this will have on his work and personal relationships, causes anxiety and stress.

The surgeon explains the nature of the operation to the patient before he gives his consent to the procedure, but a conversation with a well-informed member of the nursing staff may offer an opportunity to discuss previously undisclosed fears about the effect of surgery.

Clinical nurse specialists in mastectomy and stoma care and in other specialised branches of surgery, are experts at conveying information about the operations and may also be able to introduce the patient to someone who has experienced a similar operation and can offer advice and reassurance.

Embarrassment

Patients who depend on hearing aids, spectacles or contact lenses and dentures, suffer acute embarrassment if they are deprived of these prostheses before leaving the ward. Communication becomes increasingly difficult when they can no longer hear what is said, see what is written or formulate words coherently. These frustrations can be prevented when the nurse is aware of the problem and is prepared to use an alternative means of communication and to seek confirmation from the ward escort nurse when queries arise or to make arrangements for the removal and safe storage of these aids during the perioperative period.

The return to consciousness

Immediately before an operation fear is often expressed by the patient that he will regain consciousness during the procedure. When the anaesthetist is alerted to these apprehensions he is able to reassure the patient that he will be protected from this and similar anaesthetic hazards.

Children

Special consideration is given to the emotional problems of children coming to the operating theatre. Every effort is made to ensure that they are accompanied by someone whom they know and trust and that they are encouraged to cuddle a well-loved toy so that they are not deprived of all their familiar possessions. Preoperative preparation of these little patients usually involves looking at pictures and enacting scenes with dolls and toys to introduce the child to the clothes worn by the theatre staff and to the surroundings of the operating theatre.

Causes of stress to staff in the theatres

Working in a confined area for long periods of time and in close proximity to the other members of the team, can produce tensions and stress amongst the staff. However, when there is mutual understanding of each other's problems and needs, the tensions are dispersed and close cooperation and job satisfaction is experienced by everyone.

Noise

Harsh noises, telephone bells and shrill voices are disturbing to the sedated patient and to the surgeon and cause problems for the anaesthetist. Music is played in some theatres to induce a relaxed atmosphere.

Movement

Sudden jerky movements are liable to distract the surgeon's attention. The scrub nurse cultivates a smooth flowing rhythm when she is passing the instruments to the surgeon and she is careful not to make rapid conspicuous movements at times of intense concentration for the surgical team. Continuous traffic through the theatre doors not only increases the bacterial pollution of the theatre atmosphere but also interrupts the concentration of the surgeon.

Communication

Effective communication is of prime importance in any team activity and lack of communication causes confusion and frustration.

The scrub nurse should be in possession of all the relevant information about the patient, the operation and the procedure before the operation begins. She must give clear indications of her requirements to the other members of the team and she should inform the surgeon at the earliest possible moment if there is a problem in providing the instruments and supplies for the operation. All messages for members of the scrub team should be passed to the scrub nurse who will relay the information at a convenient moment in the procedures.

Planning and management

There is less stress amongst the theatre staff when each member of the team is given a specific job for which she is responsible and for which she has received adequate instruction to enable her to perform the task efficiently.

The team concept

The staff of the operating theatre are a closely involved team whose common aim is the provision of the best possible conditions and treatment for the patient. Each member has a clearly-defined responsibility but each person must depend on the others for support and assistance. When a good team spirit prevails there is mutual respect for the different skills of the various members and a willingness to share information. Tensions are dispelled when a good rapport and understanding exists in the team, and operations proceed in a calm and efficient atmosphere which brings job satisfaction to the staff and contributes to a safe environment for the patient.

Further reading

Boore, J (1978) A Prescription for Recovery, Royal College of Nursing Research Publications, London

Hayward, J (1975) Information—A Prescription Against Pain, Royal College of Nursing Research Publications, London

CHAPTER 4

SAFETY IN THE OPERATING DEPARTMENT

Objectives

The nurse will be able to:

1 Stipulate the precautions to take against fire and explosions in the operating department.
2 Enumerate the safeguards taken against electrical accidents and the hazards of the accumulation of static electricity in the theatre.
3 List the precautions taken to protect patients from diathermy burns.
4 Discuss the precautions taken against radiation hazards in the operating theatre.
5 Name the theatre procedure policies which safeguard the patients in the operating theatre.

Safety in the operating theatre

The purpose of the operating theatre is to provide the safest possible conditions for surgery. Safety is, therefore, the predominant consideration in the choice of design and layout of a newly-built or reconstructed department.

During the planning period, when the theatre policies are being formulated, advice is sought from experts in many fields including bacteriology, electrical and mechanical engineering and fire prevention. The finalised policy statements are used as guidelines in writing theatre procedures and channels of communication are established by which the staff will receive notice of alterations to existing procedures and details of newly-developed policies. It is the duty of the responsible persons who are nominated as safety and fire officers, to ensure that all members of the staff are familiar with the procedures for safety in the operating department.

The Health and Safety at Work Act 1974 provides legislation aimed at securing the safety of everyone at their place of work, and of any other person whose safety may be at risk by their presence in the area. The Act requires that training programmes in safety measures are planned and implemented, and stresses the importance of the individual responsibility of each person for his own safety and for the safety of others.

Instructions for the procedures to follow in emergency situations caused by fire, explosion or a major accident, are contained in hospital policy documents. All new members of staff should be given this information before they commence duties in the theatres.

Testing and checking equipment

1   Equipment must be checked each time it is to be used, and any item which does not function satisfactorily must be rejected and removed from service.

2   A clearly-written label indicating that the piece of equipment is in need of repair should be firmly attached immediately a fault is detected.

3   The problem should be communicated to the correct authority as soon as possible.

4   All repairs must be carried out by authorised persons. It is dangerous to meddle with electrical fittings and appliances. Serious accidents have occurred when inexperienced persons have undertaken repairs to vital equipment.

5   Emergency equipment must be kept ready for immediate use and checked daily.

6   Anything which appears to be out of place or unusual should be reported and investigated.

Safeguards against hazards in operating theatres

Environmental hazards

1   Regular bacteriological sampling of the air in the operating theatres.

2 The regulation of the temperature level and the relative humidity rate, to maintain optimum conditions for comfort and safety. (Temperature 22–23°C and relative humidity 55–60%.)

3 The installation of effective scavenging systems for the removal of expired anaesthetic gases.

4 Regular monitoring of the piped medical gas supply and checking the alarm signals.

5 A planned preventive maintenance programme for the ventilation and heating systems.

6 Strict observance of no smoking rules.

7 Constant checking to ensure that fire exits are unobstructed and fire doors are closed.

8 Inflammable liquids should be stored away from the vicinity of the theatres and anaesthetic rooms.

Static electricity

The static electricity which accumulates in the atmosphere presents an explosion hazard in the operating theatre. Nylon, plastics, glass, rubber and wool are liable to acquire static electricity and produce a spark when two different surfaces of these materials are rubbed together and are then separated. Serious explosions have occurred in the past when combustible substances, such as ether, were used in anaesthetics, and endoscopic lighting was supplied by heat-producing filament bulbs. The risks are greatly reduced now that the use of inflammable gases is almost discontinued and endoscopic instruments are illuminated by cold fibreoptic lights, but the risk of explosion still exists when plastic and nylon materials are used in large quantities.

Safeguards against explosions

1 Discourage the use of explosive anaesthetic agents.

2 Replace wool and nylon articles with cotton and linen.

3 Fit antistatic rubber wheels on all furniture and equipment.

4 Wear clothing of noninflammable material and footwear with antistatic substances incorporated in the sole.

5 Use anaesthetic equipment made of antistatic rubber.

6 Maintain a safe level of humidity in the operating theatre (RH 55–60%).

7 Incorporate metal conducting rods in the theatre flooring to encourage the dissipation of static electricity.

8   Never apply oil or grease to the outlets of gas cylinders. This could cause a spontaneous explosion.

Electrical hazards in the operating theatre

The installation of modern electronic machines to replace electric motors has reduced the danger of electrical accidents but discipline and caution are still required in the use of the appliances.

Safeguards against electrical accidents

1   The manufacturer's instructions for use should always be followed.
2   Cables and flexes should be sent for repair whenever breaks are detected in the wires or in the insulated covering.
3   Electric switches and sockets are placed at least three feet above ground level, where anaesthetic vapours tend to accumulate.
4   Extension cables are not used in the theatre because of the dangers from overloaded circuits, trailing flexes and sockets at ground level.
5   Special electrical sockets are fitted for use with X-ray machines that require a higher voltage than other equipment.

Electrosurgical diathermy machines

The original type of machine which produced the high frequency waves that are used to procure haemostasis during surgery was an explosive hazard in the operating theatre but the modern, solid state, transistorised unit is designed for safety and is equipped with fail safe and warning devices. (Further information on the use of electrodiathermy machines will be found in Chapter 13.)

Safeguards against accidental diathermy burns

1   Careful positioning of the indifferent electrode or patient plate to provide maximum contact between the patient's skin and the electrode.
2   The active electrode is deposited in an insulated quiver when not in use.
3   Foam rubber and padding are used to protect the patient's skin from contact with metal table attachments which could be the cause of tissue destruction when the current is in use.

4   The circulating nurse checks the dial settings with the scrub nurse and the surgeon.

Safeguards in the use and purchase of equipment

When new equipment is to be purchased the advice of experts is essential to confirm that the appliances which are selected are suitable for the purpose for which they are intended, and can be used safely with the existing equipment. Old items that are retained for further use must be evaluated frequently to ensure that the current safety standards are complied with and the government hazard warnings are observed.

Safeguards in the handling of drugs

The use and handling of scheduled poisons and controlled drugs (CD) is governed by regulations stipulated in the Poisons Rules and the Misuse of Drugs Act 1973. Each hospital establishes procedure policies for the storage, transport, administration and recording of these substances in accordance with the conditions expressed in the Rules and in the Act. The regulations issued by the hospital authorities apply to the operating department as well as in the wards and other departments, but the circumstances in the theatre usually require additional agreed policies to cover all contingencies.

Controlled and scheduled drugs are always stored in separate locked cupboards, and the keys are kept by the person in charge of the theatre who checks the contents of each container before issuing the drugs, and at the end of the session.

Injections should always be prepared by the person administering the drug and it is a necessary precaution to keep all empty ampoules and containers until the end of the operation as an identification of the substances used. Drugs, lotions and infusions should all be checked by a second person before they are poured or administered as a precaution against the mistakes which can occur in hurried and tense circumstances.

Protection against virological hazards

Isolation procedures are circulated by the control of infection committee giving directions to be followed during operations and in the disposal and

decontamination of infected material. These policies are observed whenever it is known that a patient who is coming to the operating theatre has
a high risk infection.

Safeguards against radiation hazards

Radiation hazards

The beams of image intensifier X-ray machines are more accurately
defined than those in the previously-used portable machines and a
smaller number of electrons is used on a smaller screen. The result is a
brighter picture and less radiation fallout. When X-ray exposures are to
be made in the operating theatre anyone whose presence is not
considered to be essential is advised by the radiographer to vacate the
room. The staff who remain in the area are warned to move away from
the direction of the X-ray beam and to wear lead-lined aprons to shield
their bodies from the rays.

Radioactive substances in the operating theatre

1   Policies for the handling and recording of the use of radioisotopes are
    printed and circulated by the radiology and nuclear medicine
    departments.
2   Radiation Safety Officers are responsible for the surveillance and
    implementation of protective measures.
3   An official warning notice is displayed on the door of any room in
    which there are radioisotopes.
4   Operating theatre staff are shielded from harmful rays by wearing
    protective lead aprons and using especially constructed mobile tables
    for handling exposed radioactive substances.

Further protection is afforded by maintaining a safe distance between the
source of radiation and persons in the theatre. Only those members of the
staff who are directly involved in the procedure should be allowed to
remain in the room and they are advised to keep as far away as possible
from the radium and caesium inplants.

Procedures for the protection of patients

The hospital theatre committee authorises procedures which are designed
to safeguard patients and to maintain standards of care in the operating

theatre. These procedural policies, which are periodically reviewed and amended, are presented to all the members of the staff who are responsible for their implementation. The hospital theatre policy manual usually includes guidelines on the following nursing procedures:

1   The identification of patients and checking the operation site.
2   The checking and recording of the swabs, needles and instruments used in the operation.
3   The storage, administration and recording of drugs in the operating department.
4   Procedures for aseptic techniques.
5   The collection and labelling of tissue specimens.
6   The procedure for reporting accidents in the theatre.

Services for promoting the health and safety of staff

1   In-service training in all aspects of health and safety.
2   Instruction and practice in fire prevention and fire drill.
3   Training in the application of body mechanics to prevent injuries from lifting and from prolonged standing.
4   Regular health checks at an occupational health centre. The unconscious patients in the operating theatre rely on the staff to be able to act quickly in an emergency. A high standard of fitness is required to remain alert to the possible dangers and to withstand the physical exertion and emotional tensions of theatre work. With the safety of the patient in mind, all members of the staff have a duty to report any illness or infection to the person in charge of the department, who must then decide on the course of action to be taken.

Further reading

Codes of Practice (1981) Health and Safety in Operating Theatres, National Association of Theatre Nurses

Quayle, S (1979) The Care and Safety of the Patient in the Operating Theatre, NATNews, 17: 14–16

Shaw, H (1980) Antistatic Materials and Equipment in the Operating Theatre, Surgicos Scholar Award

Reference

DHSS. Health Services Management. Health and Safety at Work Act 1974 HC (78) 30

CHAPTER 5

LEGAL AND ETHICAL ASPECTS OF OPERATING THEATRE NURSING

Objectives

The nurse will be able to:

1 Describe the circumstances that could contribute to the theatre nurse being accused of negligence.
2 List the records kept in the operating theatre.
3 Discuss the ethical aspects of operating theatre nursing.

Legal aspects of operating theatre nursing

The changes that have occurred in the operating theatres through the years have resulted in the extension of the theatre nurse's role and additional responsibilities to the patient. The nurse's job has changed from that of an assistant to that of a specialist who is responsible for her own actions. Previously, when the surgeon's role was compared to that of the captain of the ship, it was expected that he would accept responsibility for the actions of the team which directly affected patient care, but in recent years there have been increasing numbers of court cases in which theatre nurses have been called to give evidence or to answer charges of alleged professional negligence. Operating theatre nurses must, therefore, be fully aware of their individual obligations and responsibilities to the patient and the ways in which they can become involved in legal proceedings.

Definitions of legal terms

Duty

The duty of a qualified nurse is to use her knowledge and skills to maintain expected and reasonable standards of care.

Negligence

Negligence is failure to exercise the care which can be reasonably expected of a nurse in particular circumstances. To prove negligence a plaintiff must prove three things:

1 That the defendant owed him a duty of care.
2 That she was guilty of not carrying out that duty.
3 That as a result damage was caused or the plaintiff was harmed.

Responsible persons who delegate jobs to others may be accused of culpable negligence if they do not ensure that the delegated person is capable, and qualified for the task to which they are assigned.

Failure to report an incident may also amount to negligence if suffering or harm is caused as a result of the omission.

Malpractice is improper or negligent treatment by any person acting in a professional capacity.

There is a breach of duty when unreasonable risks are taken which result in injury to the patient. The nurse is responsible for her own conduct. She has the responsibility of carrying out instructions or querying them if she considers that, in her judgement, they are neither reasonable nor safe.

Informed consent to operation

It is the surgeon's duty to obtain the permission of the patient to perform an operation on him. Without this consent any operative procedure can be considered an assault or trespass on the patient's body. The law further requires that the patient must be informed of the nature of the operation, the benefits that can be reasonably expected and the possible risks involved.

The nurse's role is to check that consent has been given and that the name of the operation has been legibly written. Abbreviations for left and right and for the names of operations are not acceptable on this important document. The doctor must be informed if the patient raises queries and doubts after the form has been signed, and the problem is recorded in the nursing notes.

To obtain a valid consent the form must be signed by the patient before he receives any premedication so that he is fully aware of the conditions to which he has signified agreement.

Recording and documentation

A patient or his relatives may bring legal action for negligence long after the time of the operation. If the records are incomplete or illegible it is extremely difficult to supply the information required for legal investigation. The medical notes were, at one time, the only records giving information about the patient during the time that he was in the operating department, but many hospitals now require a continuous record of patient care throughout the perioperative period, either as part of the nursing process care plans or on the Kardex reports.

Documentation

Theatre nurses are responsible for keeping accurate and legible records which are reliable and accessible whenever they are required.

The operating theatre register

The register is used to record all the operations performed in the theatre and the names and signatures of the members of the team who were directly involved in the operation.

This book is regarded as the official record for referral whenever information is needed for legal purposes and it is, therefore, important that names and signatures are clearly written and that the record is completed promptly at the conclusion of the operation.

The controlled drugs register

A register is kept to maintain a record of the controlled drugs supplied to the department and administered to the patients.

The specimen register

Tissue and blood specimens from operations are carefully checked with the request forms, and recorded, before being transported to the laboratory for investigation.

Accident records

Hospital approved accident forms must be completed without delay whenever there is an incident or an accident involving patients or members of staff.

Safeguards against accidents at operations

The theatre nurse's duties entail constant checking with another member of the team.

The circumstances that most often cause charges of negligence to be brought against hospitals, doctors and nurses are wrong operations being performed and foreign bodies such as swabs and instruments accidently left in patients at the time of operation. The Medical Defence Union and the Royal College of Nursing issue joint memoranda with recommendations for procedures designed to prevent wrong operations being performed and the failure to remove swabs and instruments. Current editions of these booklets, which are reviewed and amended from time to time, should be available to all nurses working in operating theatres.

Ethical aspects of operating theatre nursing

Confidentiality

Nurses in the operating theatre are often in possession of information that could bring distress or cause harm if it was divulged to the wrong person. The duty of confidentiality that the nurse owes to the patient assumes even greater importance when it is remembered that she is also acting as his advocate.

Members of the operating team have an obligation to treat information about the patient which is revealed at the time of operation as strictly confidential, and to refrain from discussing the findings with other members of the staff.

The patient's notes, which may contain intimate details of his social and medical history, should be protected from scrutiny by unauthorised persons and always remain with the patient. When these documents have to be sent by messenger to another department they must be promptly despatched in a sealed envelope.

Visual display units are often used to supply computerised information to the doctors and nurses. The users of these units have a responsibility to remove the displayed data from the screen as quickly as possible, before it is witnessed by passers-by.

The dignity of the patient

Respecting the dignity of the patient and protecting him from unnecessary exposure and from actions that could cause embarrassment, are part of the nurse's duties as an advocate which are especially important when the patient is from another culture. Female patients often need to be reassured that they will be accompanied by a female nurse or doctor at all times and that they will never be left alone with male medical and nursing staff.

Transplant surgery

Transplant surgery involving the removal of tissue and organs from a cadaver or from another living body, raises controversial issues which are constantly being discussed within the medical profession and amongst the general public. Theatre nurses who assist at these procedures may have doubts and queries as to the ethical acceptance of these practices. It is important for them to read the conditions laid down in the Human Tissues Act 1961, and to be able to discuss the ethical implications with the surgeons and anaesthetists who perform these operations, and to obtain professional guidance from them.

Abortion and sterilisation

Nurses who, for religious or ethical reasons, are reluctant to assist at operations for abortion or sterilisation cannot be compelled to do so, but they have an obligation to notify the nurse in charge of the theatre of their views before they become involved in these procedures.

Research in the operating department

Research is vital for maintaining progress but there are ethical aspects to be considered, especially when patients are to be the subject of investigations in medical or nursing research. The most important factor is that the method of collecting data shall not cause distress or harm to the patient and that assurances are given that privacy and confidentiality will be respected. Participants must be fully informed of the nature of the study before consenting to information concerning them to be included in the report and they must be free to withdraw from the project at any time.

In teaching hospitals where medical research is carried out, ethical committees are appointed to assess the validity of the proposed research and to safeguard the patient from unethical practices.

Further reading

Bliss, B P and Johnson, A G (1975) Aims and Motives in Clinical Medicine, Pitman Medical

Martin, A (1977) Consent to Treatment, Nursing Times, 73: 810–811

Martin, A (1979) Confidentiality, Nursing Times, 75: 1193

Medical Defence Union and Royal College of Nursing (1983) Safeguards Against Failure to Remove Swabs and Instruments

Medical Defence Union and Royal College of Nursing (1983) Safeguards Against Wrong Operations

Young, A P (1981) Legal Problems in Nursing Practice, Harper & Row

CHAPTER 6

OPERATING THEATRE CLOTHING AND APPAREL

Objectives

The nurse will be able to:

1 Relate the history and the rationale for the development of operating theatre clothing.
2 List the criteria for the materials used in the making of theatre clothing, masks and headgear.
3 Describe the procedure for changing into theatre clothing and the disposal of used apparel.

Operating theatre clothing and apparel

History and development
At the beginning of Queen Victoria's reign surgeons wore frock coats as a mark of their professional status. The same garment was worn for ward visits and in the operating theatre, where it became caked with blood and very dirty.

If an apron was worn at all, it was for the protection of the surgeon's own clothes and with no concern for the prevention of the spread of infection. Muslin gowns were first worn during operations in 1880 after Joseph Lister had published his paper on 'The Antiseptic Principles in the Practice of Surgery', but it was not until 1920 that theatre nurses changed into special white dresses and wore cotton head coverings and face masks, whenever they entered the operating theatre.

It has now been established that the skin scales that are continually shed by everyone, carry large numbers of microbacterial organisms which will cause wound infection if they are allowed to pollute the atmosphere of the operating theatre, and the clothes that are worn in this area are designed to combat this danger. It is obligatory for all who enter the clean zone to remove outer clothing and change into special theatre garments. Convenient changing rooms and facilities are equipped with lockers in which to hang outer garments to keep them separate from those worn in the theatre. The choice of material, design and colour varies in each hospital, but certain criteria are established to guide those responsible for ordering and supplying theatre clothing.

Design

Originally, dresses only were worn by the female staff but since the realisation that there is a high degree of bacterial fallout from the perineum, trousers and pantsuits have become accepted as the most suitable wear for both men and women (Figure 6.1).

1 Ribbed cuffs or press fastenings ensure a close fit around the ankles.
2 Simple, straight tunic shapes are less hazardous than swirling hems and baggy trousers where there are sterile trolleys and tables to be avoided.
3 Sleeves are cut short to end well above the elbow and will not interfere with the scrubbing-up procedure.
4 Fastenings must be easy to adjust and able to withstand repeated laundering without becoming lost or broken.

Manufacturers are continually striving to produce designs that are smart and tidy, allow unrestricted movement and are acceptable to all the personnel in the operating theatres.

Materials

Fabric requirements

1 Close woven to prevent skin scales and dust from escaping into the atmosphere.
2 Durable and easily laundered.
3 Light in weight and lint free.

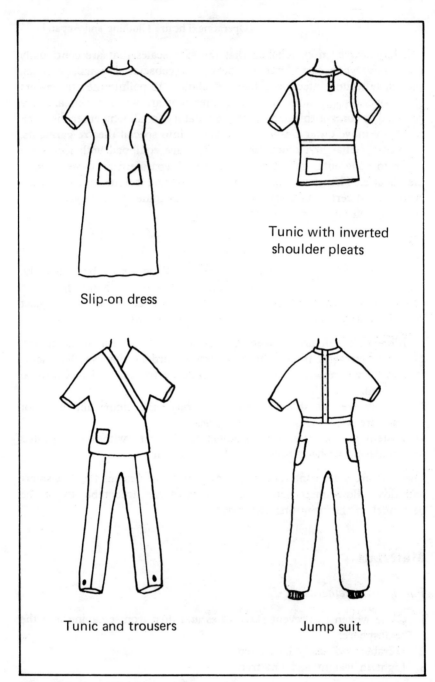

Slip-on dress

Tunic with inverted
shoulder pleats

Tunic and trousers

Jump suit

Figure 6.1 Operating theatre dresses and suits.

Cotton-polyester is often the fabric of choice because this mixture of man-made and natural fibres fulfils the above requirements and reduces the risk of accumulated static electricity.

Colour

Plain colours are preferred in some hospitals but pretty patterns and attractive colour combinations are also available.

Head Coverings

It is imperative that all hair is covered in the operating theatre because human hair is the source of a large proportion of the bacterial particles that pervade the atmosphere. A choice of caps, helmets and turbans is provided to accommodate all kinds of hair styles for both men and women.

The material used for head coverings is:

1 Non-woven to prevent the seepage of bacterial particles.
2 Lint free.
3 Light in weight.
4 Easily disposed of.

Coloured and flowered caps are often worn as a convenient means of identifying different grades of staff.

Materials for face masks

The face mask is intended to filter the exhaled breath of the wearer and must fit snugly around the bridge of the nose, the sides of the face and under the chin. Face masks are produced in a standard size that is adapted to fit various facial shapes by using adjustable or elastic head tapes, pleated material and malleable metal strips that fit over the nose.

1 The material must ensure efficient bacterial filtration of the moisture-laden expired air for the duration of an operation.
2 Materials must be lint free and non-allergenic to the wearer.
3 Disposable synthetic materials are the most effective.
4 The packaging must allow each mask to be removed from the container by the tapes to eliminate handling and contamination of the face piece.

Footwear

Wellington boots, clogs and canvas shoes are suitable forms of footwear for the operating theatre provided that antistatic material is incorporated in the sole. The shoes require testing at regular intervals to confirm that the antistatic properties are retained.

Sandals and light shoes that do not give adequate protection from injury are a safety hazard to staff in the operating theatre.

Preparation for entering the operating theatre

Personal hygiene is important. Hair and skin must be scrupulously clean and any abrasions or infected lesions should be reported to the nurse in charge of the theatre. Showers increase the rate at which skin particles are shed and should not be taken immediately before going into the operating theatre.

Jewellery is a hazard when worn in the theatre. Bacterial shedding is increased by the friction of metal or abrasive material in contact with skin, and there are added dangers to the patient:

1 Ear-rings can become dislodged and fall into the wound.
2 Chains and necklaces become entangled in the patient's clothing.
3 Rings harbour dirt and dust particles and cause skin abrasions during positioning procedures.

The procedure for personnel entering the clean zone

The order of dressing should conform to a routine that diminishes the danger of contaminating clean clothing by contact with outer clothes.

1 Remove outer clothing and hang in a locker or a designated space.
2 Put on a theatre cap or head-covering. Check in the mirror that the hair is completely covered.
3 Remove all jewellery. (Plain gold band wedding rings are usually permitted to be worn.)
4 Remove heavy make-up.
5 Wash your hands.
6 Select and don appropriate clothing.
7 Step into theatre shoes at the clean zone barrier.

Wearing a face mask

1 Take a mask from the container before entering the sterile area. Handle the tapes and the edges only.

2 Mould the mask to fit around the nose.
3 Tie the tapes. Upper tapes passed over the ears and tied at the back of the head; lower tapes tied at the back of the neck.
4 Discard used masks after each operation or on leaving the theatre.
5 Do not wear masks hanging from the neck.
6 Used masks should not be handled or stored in pockets.

The disposal of used theatre apparel

1 Remove the mask outside the operating theatre. Handling the tapes only, drop the mask into a disposal bin.
2 Remove shoes at the changing room barrier or shoe rack.
3 Remove and dispose of headgear.
4 Place used clothing in the nearest linen bin.
5 Wash your hands before dressing in outer clothes.

In the future, when durable and comfortable non-woven fabric is produced more cheaply, theatre personnel will probably be able to wear disposable apparel, but the individual responsibility of conscientiously following procedures that reduce the risk of infection will remain.

Further reading

Coombes, B (1978) The Importance of Being Well Dressed in Theatre, NATNews, 15: 6–8

CHAPTER 7

ASEPTIC TECHNIQUES

Objectives

The nurse will be able to:

1 Identify the techniques employed to preserve asepsis and prevent the spread of infection in the operating theatre.
2 List the methods used for the sterilisation of surgical instruments and equipment.
3 Describe the procedure for the disposal of used materials at the end of an operation.

Development of aseptic techniques

Infection occurs when bacteria enter the body, multiply and produce a reaction. The bacteria cling to dust particles and may be carried into the operating theatre by air currents and people, on solid objects or in liquids. When the bacteria contaminate the surgical wound and cause infection to develop, the patient suffers pain, healing is delayed and convalescence is prolonged.

Lord Joseph Lister is known as the father of antiseptic surgery. In 1867 he published a paper in the British Medical Journal entitled 'The Antiseptic Principle in the Practice of Surgery'. Lister sprayed the wound and the surrounding areas with phenol to destroy bacteria and prevent them from invading the patient's body tissues. His theories laid the foundation for the development of modern aseptic techniques and the basic principles established by Lister still apply today. In recent years the development of chemotherapy and antibiotics has dramatically reduced the incidence of wound infection, but conscientious use of aseptic procedures, by all the members of the surgical team, is a vitally important factor in the prevention of the spread of infection in the operating theatre.

Principles of aseptic technique

The following basic aseptic techniques are used to prevent the transfer of bacteria to the operating theatre.

Environmental

1 Regular house-keeping and cleaning programmes are instigated and constantly reviewed to assess the efficiency of the methods and materials employed.
2 Routine bacteriological sampling tests of floors and furniture are carried out.
3 The prevention of dust accumulation.
4 Positive pressure ventilation to provide rapid removal of contaminants from the atmosphere.
5 Keeping the doors closed and avoidance of unnecessary movement.

Non-scrubbed personnel

1 Admission to the operating theatre is restricted to those persons whose presence is necessary.
2 Conversation is kept to a minimum to prevent droplet bacterial spread.
3 Operating theatre clothing is worn by all who enter the clean zone.
4 Persons who are not scrubbed and wearing sterile gowns and gloves must avoid stretching or leaning over sterile trolleys and tables and keep a reasonable and safe distance from sterile surfaces, to avoid contaminating them.

Scrubbed personnel

1 Gowns are considered to be sterile only on the front, from waist to shoulder level, and the sleeves, i.e. the areas that may come in contact with the drapes covering the sterile field.

2   Gloved hands are protected from contamination by holding the hands, palms together, above waist level.
3   All scrubbed members of the surgical team remain within the operating theatre throughout the operation.
4   When it is necessary for two members of the scrubbed team to change places they should pass either back to back or front to front.

The preparation of sterile trolleys and tables

1   Tables and trolleys are considered to be sterile, only at table height and above.
2   When opening sterile packs the scrub nurse drapes an unsterile trolley or table by first covering the near side, drawing the drapes towards her, and then the far side.
3   Sterile handling forceps are used by the scrub nurse to extract wrapped items from sterile packets so that the circulating nurse does not risk holding her hands over the sterile trolley or shaking dust on to the sterile field.
4   All sterile surfaces are kept dry to prevent bacterial seepage through moist linen.
5   Sterile trolleys should be prepared immediately before they are to be used.
6   If there is any doubt at all regarding the sterility of an item to be used in an operation, it is discarded.

Circulating nurse

1   Sealed sterile packets are opened with care so that the contents do not come into contact with the unsterile outer edges of the package or with ungloved hands.
2   Any package that is dropped on the floor will be contaminated and must be discarded.
3   Sterile packets are inspected before they are opened to confirm that the wrappings are intact and undamaged.
4   Lotions are poured into bowls held away from the sterile field or placed at the outer edge of the trolley so that the circulating nurse's ungloved hands are not held over the sterile area.

Sterilisation

Sterilisation means the destruction of all known micro-organisms. It is an absolute quality and there can be no degrees of sterility.

Many of the commodities used at an operation are prepackaged and sterilised commercially. These disposable items are intended to be used once only and should not be resterilised. Reusable articles are prepared centrally in a Theatre Sterile Supply Unit (TSSU) by personnel who are experienced in packaging and sterilising techniques or in the operating theatre by members of the theatre team.

Principles of sterilisation (Table 7.1)

1 The article to be sterilised must be clean. Deposits of blood, mucus and grease prevent the sterilising agent from making direct contact with all surfaces.
2 The sterilising process must be suitable, reliable, and proved to be efficient.

Table 7.1 Summary of the principle methods of sterilisation used in operating theatres

Sterilising method	Temperature	Time
1 High prevacuum steriliser Steam pressure Pulsing Drying phase	134°C	3 min
2 Downward displacement steriliser Steam pressure No drying phase	134°C	3 min
3 Low temperature steam and formaldehyde Subatmospheric pressure Steam Formaldehyde	72–80°C	1–2 h
4 Ethylene oxide Moisture and carbon dioxide Low temperature Requires aeration period of 24 hours	50°C	1–16 h
5 Hot air oven	160°C	1 h

3   The method of preparation and packaging that is employed should allow the article to be delivered to the sterile field without coming into contact with ungloved hands.
4   Wrapped articles must be packaged in materials that comply with the specifications of the DHSS to withstand the sterilising process and to effectively resist the penetration of dust during storage.

The physical and chemical properties of each item have to be assessed before a particular method of sterilisation is selected. Steam under pressure is considered to be the most effective means of destroying bacteria and spores but instruments and equipment made of materials that are heat and moisture sensitive must be sterilised by other methods. The manufacturer's instructions should always be consulted before sterilising new and specialised equipment.

Physical methods of sterilisation

1   Steam under pressure.
2   Dry heat. Hot air ovens.
3   Ionising radiation. Gamma rays.

Chemical methods of sterilisation

1   Formaldehyde gas with low temperature steam at subatmospheric pressure.
2   Ethylene oxide gas.

Sterilisation by steam under pressure

This is the method most widely used in hospitals. There is no toxic residue, the steam and heat that are produced are easily controlled and the process is not expensive. The machines that are used for sterilisation by this means are complex and costly and have been highly developed for maximum efficiency.

High prevacuum sterilisers or autoclaves

These modern and automatically-operated machines provide the most effective method for sterilising porous loads of linen and instruments used in the operating theatre.

Components of an autoclave steriliser

The chamber is a steel-lined oven with reinforced doors that are operated by an electric motor. The jacket is an outer casing of steel which surrounds the chamber leaving a gap of approximately one inch between the chamber wall and the outer jacket. The space is filled with steam at a constant pressure of 15 lb/in^2 to prevent loss of heat from the chamber wall and to assist the drying process.

Charts, dials and gauges record the temperature and pressure attained and the time taken for each stage of the cycle. Adequate supplies of steam, water and electricity must be available.

Suitable loads for high prevacuum sterilisers

1 Porous materials. Linen, paper and materials that will withstand moisture and a temperature of 134°C.
2 Instruments and bowls packaged in paper or freshly-laundered linen.
3 Instruments and bowls that are unwrapped and loaded in wire trays.

Stages of the sterilising cycle (Figure 7.1)

1 Loading. The steriliser is loaded with the heaviest packs of metal instruments on the lower shelf.
2 Cycle start. When the cycle start switch is operated the doors are closed and sealed.
3 Pulsing. Steam is pumped into the chamber and mixes with the residual air. The mixture of air and steam is then withdrawn by a vacuum pump. This process is repeated until a vacuum of 30 in Hg (inches of mercury) is obtained in the chamber and all the residual air has been removed from the steriliser and the contents.
4 Vacuum. When a vacuum has been drawn, steam is admitted to the chamber and penetrates all of the load until a maximum pressure of 32 lb/in^2 is attained and a uniform temperature of 134°C is recorded.
5 Sterilising. These conditions are maintained for 3 to 4 minutes to ensure the destruction of all micro-organisms.
6 Drying. Steam and moisture are withdrawn from the chamber and the load by a pumping system which draws a vacuum of 25 in Hg. The heat generated from the steam jacket aids the drying process.
7 Process end. When the drying time is completed, bacteria-filtered air is injected into the chamber to restore the pressure within to normal atmospheric pressure, and then the door can safely be opened and the steriliser unloaded. Sterile packets should be left to cool on a rack for at least 15 minutes after unloading.

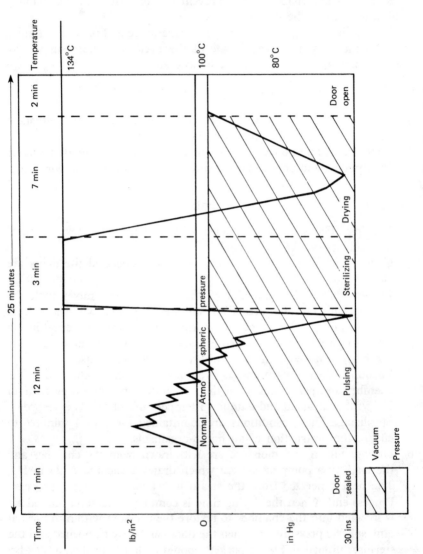

Figure 7.1   Stages of the sterilising cycle in a high prevacuum steriliser. Porous load.

The entire sterilising process is completed in 25 minutes. If the optimum conditions have not been maintained during the cycle a 'Not Sterile' indicator appears on the switch panel and the door remains closed, to eliminate the risk of using articles that have not been successfully sterilised.

Downward displacement gravity sterilisers

These autoclaves are similar in design to the high prevacuum steriliser and can produce a temperature of 134°C within the chamber.

Air in the chamber is removed by the gravity displacement of air by steam. When steam, which is lighter than air, is injected from above, the air is forced through an outlet drain in the floor of the chamber. There is no provision for a pulsing phase to remove residual air from tubing and porous materials and there is no drying phase.

Suitable loads for downward displacement sterilisers

1   Unwrapped bowls and instruments.
2   Non-porous items able to withstand heat and moisture.
3   Laboratory utensils and fluids in sealed containers.

Stages of the cycle

1   The chamber is loaded.
2   The door is closed and sealed.
3   Steam is admitted until the load reaches a temperature of 134°C. A timer is energised to maintain these conditions for 3 to 4 minutes.
4   Venting. The chamber is evacuated of steam and moisture by a pump, to produce a vacuum of 25 in Hg.
5   Air injection. Air is admitted to the chamber until normal atmospheric pressure prevails inside the steriliser.
6   Process end. The doors are opened and the load is removed.

Hot air oven sterilisers

Dry heat is employed when the use of steam is inappropriate. The temperature in an electrically heated oven is raised slowly and must circulate to all surfaces for even distribution. The temperature in the oven is recorded throughout the sterilising process and the air is circulated by fans.

Suitable loads

1   Petroleum jelly, oil and fats that resist penetration by steam.
2   Fine cutting instruments and articles that can be damaged by moisture.

The prolonged slow exposure to heat is harmful to cloth materials and rubber.

The sterilising process

1   The oven is loaded allowing sufficient space between the items for the hot air to circulate.
2   The temperature of the entire load is raised slowly to 160°C.
3   Hot air circulates continuously to maintain this temperature in all parts of the oven for 60 minutes.
4   At process end the load is allowed to cool slowly before removal from the oven.

Gamma ray ionising radiation

Gamma rays are commercially used for the sterilisation of prepackaged goods used in the operating theatre. The rays of the radioisotope cobalt 60 are used in a large, especially-constructed plant and the packets are exposed to the rays while they move along on a conveyor belt.

Suitable loads

1   Prepackaged items in foil or plastic film.
2   Disposable hypodermic needles and syringes.
3   Catheters.
4   Blades and sharp instruments.

Gamma rays can cause deterioration and chemical changes in some substances, particularly if they have been sterilised previously. The manufacturers instructions concerning resterilising that are on the packaging of items sterilised by gamma rays must be followed.

Formaldehyde with low temperature steam at subatmospheric pressure

A high prevacuum steriliser is modified to use steam at subatmospheric pressure and a temperature that is controlled at 70–80°C for sterilising heat-sensitive articles. Formalin is injected into the steam in measured amounts to produce a concentration of formaldehyde.

Suitable loads

1 Reusable instruments and equipment that cannot withstand temperatures above 70–80°C without sustaining damage or destruction.
2 Cystoscopes and endoscopic instruments that are unwrapped or packaged in paper or transparent film.

Linen will absorb the gas, thereby reducing the concentration of formaldehyde.

Stages of the cycle
The steriliser is loaded, allowing space between the packages.

1 Pulsing. When the cycle start switch is activated the doors are closed and sealed and steam is introduced into the chamber where it mixes with the residual air and is then withdrawn by a vacuum pump. This process is repeated until a vacuum of 25 in Hg and a temperature of 72°C is produced. Formalin is injected into the chamber during the pulsing phase to maintain a measured concentration of gas.
2 Sterilising. The load is exposed to formaldehyde gas under these conditions for one hour.
3 Drying process and removal of formaldehyde. The chamber is evacuated by a pulsing action which reduces the vacuum and removes the formaldehyde and the moisture.
4 Filtered air is admitted to the chamber to equalise the pressure in the chamber with that of the normal atmosphere.
5 The door is opened and the packages removed.

Ethylene oxide gas

Ethylene oxide gas is frequently used commercially for the sterilising of heat-resistant articles such as those made of PVC and petrochemical substances. When ethylene oxide is used in hospitals, especially designed machines are required for use with the cylinders of highly explosive gas. Stringent safety precautions must be followed to protect the steriliser operators and to eliminate the residual gas from the sterilised items because ethylene oxide, and its byproducts, are very toxic and irritant to skin and mucous membrane.

Sterilisation by ethylene oxide requires a relative humidity of 30% in the chamber.

Suitable loads

Articles must be packaged in gas-permeable wrappings.

1 Cardiac catheters and pacemakers.
2 Arterial grafts.
3 PVC and plastic materials.
4 Respiratory and anaesthetic equipment.
5 Electrical equipment.
6 Suture material.

Stages of the cycle

1 Vacuum. Air is withdrawn from the chamber and a vacuum of 25 in Hg is created.
2 Humidifying. A regulated relative humidity of 30–40% is produced in the chamber and the moisture permeates the contents of the load.
3 Sterilising. Ethylene oxide (10%) and 90% carbon dioxide or a similar mixture of gases is injected into the chamber. The sterilising time varies from 2½ to 5 hours depending on the packaging used and the type of load.
4 Drying and air flushing. The gas is evacuated by drawing a vacuum of 25 in Hg. Air is admitted and withdrawn by a pulsing action to reduce the gas concentration.
5 Process end. Filtered air enters the chamber until normal atmospheric pressure prevails and the door can be opened.
6 Aeration period. It is essential to allow an aeration period of at least 24 hours to elapse before using the sterilised articles.

Steriliser controls and tests

The Bowie-Dick test is designed to test for the successful removal of air from the chamber and the contents of a porous load cycle in a high prevacuum steriliser. The test should be performed daily, before the first sterilising cycle of the day, and the results must be retained and recorded for future reference.

The Bowie-Dick daily test for high prevacuum sterilisers

Method:

1 Clean, dry huckaback towels (British Standard 1781 TLS) size 36 × 24 inches, are each folded into eight thicknesses. The towels are placed one above the other to form a pile 10 to 11 inches high. Twenty five to thirty towels will be required.

2 A square of sterilising paper, 12 inches square, bearing a cross of 3M Autoclave indicator tape is placed in the centre of the pile of towels.

3 The towels are secured in a sheet or wrapper and placed in the centre of an empty steriliser. The porous load cycle is started.

4 At the end of the cycle, the test paper is removed from the pile and inspected. The coloured stripes of the autoclave tape should be the same colour at the centre of the cross as at the outside edges.

5 If the stripes on the tape are of uniform colour, the unit is ready for use provided that the charts record that the temperature attained in the chamber and the length of sterilising time is satisfactory.

Air leak test

Tests are carried out regularly by steriliser operators or engineers to detect air leaking into the chamber through a faulty valve or door seal of high vacuum sterilisers.

Chemical indicator tests

Heat-sensitive chemicals which change colour when subjected to heat, are supplied in small sealed tubes which can be incorporated in normal sterilising loads to indicate that the process was satisfactory.

Indicator tubes can be obtained for testing:

1 Hot air ovens.
2 Downward displacement sterilisers.
3 High prevacuum sterilisers.

Microbiological tests

Strips of heat-resistant spores are placed in test packs or normal sterilising loads, and are then cultured in the laboratory to determine whether the spores have been destroyed in the sterilising process.

Autoclave indicator tape

Adhesive tape that is used to secure the outer wrapping of packets will develop dark brown stripes after being submitted to heat in a sterilising process.

Colour indicator disc

A yellow disc on the packaging of goods exposed to gamma rays, turns red during the sterilising process.

Materials used for packaging

Cotton cloth

The material must be closely woven with 140 threads to the square inch and freshly laundered each time it is used. The three layers that are required to preserve the sterility of the contents of the packet are provided by a single thickness inner sheet and a double thickness wrapper for the outer layer.

Paper

Paper used for packaging must comply with the specifications issued by the DHSS. Two layers of paper, or one sheet of paper and an outer bag, are required to protect the sterile contents and to facilitate the removal of the article without risk of contamination by contact with the outer surface of the packet. The paper must be folded in such a manner that, as the packet is unfolded, any dust particles that are present will fall outwards away from the sterile article. This is most satisfactorily achieved by folding in an envelope fashion.

Nylon film

Nylon film bags are manufactured in convenient sizes. The material is strong and provides adequate protection but it is easily punctured by sharp objects and is most suitable for the packaging of small light articles.

Non-woven materials

Disposable synthetic materials that have properties that are comparable to those required for cotton or paper may be used for sterilisation packaging.

Paper bags

Paper bags must be made of Kraft paper and the seams sealed with two lines of strong adhesive. They are made in various sizes with an adequate gusset to allow the contents to be easily withdrawn. The outside of the packet is clearly labelled with an exact description of the contents, date stamped and sealed by an effective roller heat-sealer or by folding the top edges over three times and securing each corner with autoclave indicator tape.

Marking pencils

Sharp pointed pens and spirit-based markers produce small perforations in the paper but soft chinagraph pencils do not damage the packaging and remain unchanged by heat and moisture in the sterilising process.

Immersion in chemical solutions

Some chemical solutions are capable of destroying all micro-organisms, including spores, provided that the instrument is left in contact with the sterilising agent for the requisite length of time, as stated by the manufacturer. This method should only be used when alternative means are unavailable because there is no biological test that the user can employ to prove sterility and there are hazards to overcome to ensure that the instruments have not been recontaminated when they are delivered to the sterile field. Immersion in a chemical solution cannot be classified, therefore, as a reliable and acceptable sterilising method.

Hazards in the use of chemical solutions

1 The solution must be in contact with all surfaces of the instrument for the recommended length of time. Tubular or cannulated instruments, such as cystoscope sheaths, must stand upright in the container to avoid an air bubble preventing the solution from reaching all of the lumen.
2 The instrument must be dry. Any moisture added to the solution will cause dilution and render the agent ineffective.
3 Lifting the instrument out of the solution at the end of the allocated time must be accomplished without touching the outside walls of the container.
4 Thorough rinsing is essential to remove all traces of the irritant chemical agent from the instrument.

Pasteurisation

This is a disinfecting process that will destroy some vegetative bacteria.

Delicate instruments, like telescopes and cystoscopes, are immersed in a bath of water at a temperature of 70°C for ten minutes.

The disposal of used equipment following an operation

All items that have come into contact with the patient or the sterile field, are regarded as contaminated and are removed by a separate route which will ensure that dirty, used articles do not come into contact with unused sterile packs and equipment. A conscientious approach to the safe disposal and cleaning of items used in surgery will prevent:

1   The spread of infection by contamination.
2   Injury to handling personnel.
3   Loss or damage to equipment.
4   Delays in the recycling of instruments and equipment.

At the end of the operation

1   Patient drapes are removed by the scrub nurse with gloved hands.
2   All used and soiled linen is despatched to the laundry in sealed bags.
3   Disposable items are collected with other rubbish and sealed in a plastic bag.
4   Gowns and gloves worn by the scrubbed members of the team are removed and deposited in plastic-lined containers within the operating theatre.
5   Bowls and instruments are collected and sent to the cleaning and disposal room or to the TSSU to be washed in detergent solution.
6   Knife blades are removed from handles by the scrub nurse and safely deposited with the opened, disposable, needles in a sealed container.
7   Hypodermic needles and syringes are disposed of in strong sealed boxes.
8   Aerosol cannisters, that are dangerous when incinerated, are collected for safe disposal.
9   Lotions and suction jar contents are flushed away in a sluice.
10   All solid surfaces are cleaned with disinfectant solution.

Disinfection following high risk infected cases

When an operation is to be performed on a patient with a known specific infection, such as serum hepatitus, all the furniture and equipment that will not be used during the operation is removed from the theatre. A second circulating nurse is positioned outside the theatre door to fetch extra supplies and to relay messages for the staff inside the theatre.

The use of disposables, that can be destroyed without further handling, reduces the hazards to the theatre staff and porters and lessens the risk of the spread of infection. Disposable aprons, gowns and shoe covers are issued to all personnel who will be in the theatre during the operation. Protective goggles can be issued to the scrubbed members of the team.

Admission to the operating theatre is restricted to those persons whose presence is necessary for the operation to proceed. It is not permissible to leave the theatre and return again, except by using the 'dirty route' for used items, which necessitates shedding shoe covers and outer gowns.

Blood or pus that is spilt on the floor or the walls should be covered immediately with a germicide solution before it is wiped away, and all persons handling contaminated or used articles should wear protective gloves.

At the end of the operation

1 All personnel leave the theatre by the disposal route and discard shoe coverings, caps, gowns and masks in the dirty utility area.
2 Instruments and reusable items that will withstand heat and moisture should, if possible, be autoclaved before they are washed.
3 Disposable knife blades and needles should be autoclaved before disposal.
4 Sealed bags of rubbish must bear a hazard label and be destroyed by incineration without delay.
5 Thorough disinfection of the theatre must be completed before operating can be recommenced.

A cleaning procedure approved by the microbiologist and the control of infection committee must be conscientiously followed. The procedure should give instructions in the use of disinfectants, the length of time to elapse before reuse, and any microbiological tests that are required.

Further reading

Parker, M and Stucke, V (1982) Microbiology for Nurses, 6th edition, Nurses Aids Series, Baillière Tindall
Smith, A (1973) Principles of Microbiology, Mosby

CHAPTER 8

THE PATIENT'S ARRIVAL IN THE OPERATING DEPARTMENT

Objectives

The nurse will be able to:

1 Describe the procedure for checking the identity and the preoperative preparation of the patient for surgery.
2 Enumerate the safety measures that are employed for the protection of the patient in the reception area.
3 Identify potential patient problems and develop plans for providing a continuity of nursing care in the operating theatre.

The reception of patients

The reception of patients when they arrive in the operating theatre prior to surgery, is one of the most important duties performed by the theatre staff. It is at this time that the theatre nurse accepts the responsibility, as the patient's advocate, of acting on his behalf and guarding his safety during the period of sedation and anaesthesia.

In the reception area, where responsibility for the care of the patient is transferred from the ward nurse to the operating theatre staff, a quiet and calm atmosphere is reassuring to the apprehensive patient. Emotional stress, which is often experienced immediately before an operation, can be alleviated by a word of encouragement and a welcoming smile from the receiving nurse as she introduces herself to the patient.

Identification

The nurse asks the patient to say his own name and checks that the name and number that is shown on his identification label corresponds with those on the accompanying medical records and the operating list.

Consent to operation

The receiving nurse confirms that the patient has signed the form giving his consent to the operation. The escorting nurse is asked to assist with the checking procedure, particularly when the patient is asleep or unable to communicate, due to a hearing or speech defect.

Premedication

The time of the administration of the prescribed premedication is checked, and any adverse reaction is reported to the anaesthetist without delay.

Preoperative preparation

A check list is a useful guide to the receiving nurse in establishing that the preparation for anaesthesia and surgery has been satisfactorily completed.

Preoperative preparation check list

1 The patient's skin is clean and the operation site has been prepared.
2 The site of operation is clearly marked on the patient's skin.
3 The time of the last food and fluid intake has been recorded.
4 The time of voiding of the bladder.
5 A catheter is in situ.
6 Jewellery and hair pins have been removed.
7 A wedding ring, if worn, has been secured with adhesive tape.
8 Contact lenses or spectacles have been removed.
9 Dentures have been removed.
10 Crowned and loose teeth have been recorded.
11 The wearing of a hearing aid is noted and reported. Hearing aids that have been removed may be lodged in the recovery room until the patient recovers consciousness.
12 The position of implanted prosthesis is noted.
13 Known allergies are recorded.

14 The patients records are complete:
   a Medical records.
   b X-ray and laboratory reports.
   c Nursing history.
   d Nursing care plans or Kardex.

When this procedure has been completed, the escorting nurse takes her leave of the patient who is transferred to a theatre trolley and accompanied to the anaesthetic room.

Patient safety

Theatre staff are always aware of the potential dangers to patients at the transfer area and the necessity to remain alert and ready to protect the patient from harm.

Guidelines for patient safety

1   The patient is never left alone in the operating theatre department.
2   All records must be legibly written, dated and signed.
3   Abbreviations are not acceptable on recording documents.
4   Stretcher canvases used for transporting patients must be inspected to confirm that they are intact and safe.
5   The patient is positioned on the canvas with adequate support for head and limbs.
6   The wheels of trolleys are securely locked before attempting to transfer the patient.
7   Retaining side rails are raised and secured before the trolley is moved.
8   The nurse stands at the far side of the receiving trolley to support and assist the patient.
9   Intravenous infusions are guarded by the nurse during transfer.

Nursing care plans

A nursing history of each patient is recorded, on the day of his admission to the ward, in the hospital where the nursing process is implemented. Past and present medical records and a social history, which are included in these notes, are reviewed by the theatre nurse when she is assessing the patient's needs. Additional information can be gathered during a preoperative visit to the patient in the ward. This interview gives the patient an opportunity to meet a nurse who will care for him in the operating theatre and who can explain the procedures at the reception area. While they converse, the theatre nurse may detect signs of anxiety and tension that can be dispelled by explaining the reasons for the preoperative preparations and discussing plans for alleviating problems that are caused by physical disabilities.

Observations

When circumstances do not allow a preoperative visit to be made, an assessment of the patient's needs must be formulated from the information contained in the nursing history and from observations made by the receiving nurse when the patient arrives in the operating department.

The observation of patients

1   General appearance—satisfactory, emaciated, thin, obese.
2   Skin colour—normal, pale, flushed, cyanosed.
3   Skin condition:
    a   Normal, dehydrated, oedematous.
    b   Intact, broken, rash, blemishes.
4   Mobility—agile, stiff joints, paralysis.
5   Emotional state:
    a   Orientated, confused, anxious.
    b   Cheerful, composed, morose, unresponsive.

Stages in the preparation of care plans

1   Assessment. Present a clear statement of each problem that is identified by observation and the collection of data from the nursing history.
2   Establishment of a goal. State the goal, objective or expected outcome set by the nurse for the patient.
3   Planning. Describe the plans that are formulated, state who will perform the action and when it will occur.
4   Implementation. Perform and record the proposed actions.
5   Evaluation. Evaluate the outcome of the recorded nursing care.

Guidelines in the use of care plans

The plans should be:

1   Clearly written and concise.
2   Easily accessible at all times.

	Problem	Goal	Plan	Implementation	Evaluation
1	Patient is deaf and lip-reads. She is afraid she will not be able to follow spoken instructions	The patient will be able to see the mouths of all theatre staff to lip-read and will be reassured and relaxed.	Warn the receiving nurse to face patient and speak clearly. Receiving nurse to alert anaesthetic and recovery room staff to problem.	Receiving nurse conversed with patient. Anaesthetic room staff removed masks and faced patient. At end of case anaesthetic room staff alerted recovery room staff to problem.	Patient relaxed and reassured. Able to follow instructions. Recovery uneventful. Patient very grateful for help and consideration.
2	Patient has stiff right knee for which she has physiotherapy. She is concerned that positioning for a D & C will cause pain and further damage.	There will be no undue postoperative pain or immobility of right knee.	Problem to be discussed with theatre sister. Staff nurse to supervise positioning on operating table.	Staff nurse lifted patient's right knee during positioning. Stirrup adjusted to prevent over-extension.	No postoperative pain and patient able to walk on following day.

Figure 8.1 Nursing care plans.

3   Referred to frequently by nursing staff.
4   Evaluated and reviewed.
5   A continuous record of nursing care.

Recording care plans

Care plans provide a written record of the stages in a systematic approach to nursing care (Figure 8.1). Goals or objectives are set by which the effect of the treatment can be evaluated after the operation. The method of recording information and communicating the plans to the operating team will vary in each hospital. A separate duplicated sheet for recording the plans and the care given in the theatre department has been used with success in some hospitals. One copy of the record sheet is filed with the patient's notes and the second copy is lodged in the theatre department, where it is available for all the members of the team to read before making the preparations for each individual patient.

In order to show a continuous record of care the format used on the surgical wards can be adapted for writing theatre care plans.

The establishment of a successful and acceptable means of gathering the necessary data requires good liaison with the surgical ward nurses and offers opportunities for the exchange of knowledge and ideas that lead to improvements in patient care.

Further reading

Gruendemann, B J (1977) The Surgical Patient. Behavioural Concepts for the Operating Room Nurse, Mosby

CHAPTER 9

THE NURSE IN THE ANAESTHETIC ROOM

Objectives

The nurse will be able to:

1 Enumerate the types of anaesthesia and analgesia used for surgery.
2 Describe the equipment used for the induction and maintenance of anaesthesia.
3 Describe the preparation of the anaesthetic room and the reception of the patient.
4 Outline the anaesthetic nurse's duties and responsibilities.
5 List the complications that can arise during anaesthesia.

The development of surgical anaesthesia

Extracts from herbs and plants have been used since the earliest ages of man to induce sleep and to remove the sensations of pain but surgical anaesthesia was not developed until the middle of the nineteenth century.

At first, ether and chloroform vapours were used but the primitive methods of administration employed at that time delivered high concentrations of these drugs and caused severe vomiting and nausea. Many of the casualties in the First World War had facial injuries and needed intubation to enable them to inhale anaesthetic gases during the long plastic surgery operations, and in 1942 the use of muscle relaxant drugs reduced the risks and introduced the concept of balanced anaesthesia. In recent years anaesthesia has been rendered safer and more reliable by improvements in equipment, advances in pharmacology and the development of sophisticated machinery for the monitoring of the patient's reactions.

Operating theatre nurses in the anaesthetic room

In the first operating theatres the escort nurse from the surgical ward accompanied the patient to the anaesthetic room and stayed with him during the induction of the anaesthetic. Nowadays many of our modern hospitals appoint anaesthetic staff to care for the patient and to assist the anaesthetist, but every operating theatre nurse should acquire a knowledge of anaesthetic procedures to enable her to fulfil the commitment to give nursing care throughout the entire perioperative period.

Types of analgesia and anaesthesia

Local analgesia

Analgesia means the absence of pain. Local or regional analgesia is induced by the application or injection of drugs in order to interrupt the pathway of the sensory nerves from the area.

Topical analgesia

A solution of the drug is applied to the skin or mucous membrane to produce analgesia of the area and to reduce discomfort during procedures of short duration.

Methods of application

1 The solution is sprayed directly on to the surface of the throat and nasal passages.
2 Ointment containing an analgesic is applied to the urethra.
3 Drops containing the drug in solution are inserted in the eye.

The agents most commonly used for these procedures are cocaine, lignocaine and amethocaine.

Infiltration analgesia

An analgesic agent is injected at several points over the operation site. The solution infiltrates the tissues around the nerve endings in the skin to remove the sensation of pain during minor surgical procedures.

Field block

The drug is introduced as for infiltration but the injections are sited at several points surrounding the operation area. Field blocks can be used satisfactorily for abdominal operations when general anaesthesia is contraindicated.

Nerve block

A solution of the analgesic is injected around the main nerve which supplies the tissues involved in the operation. Nerve blocks are a convenient means of producing analgesia of limbs and extremities.

Spinal nerve analgesia

Spinal analgesia entails the introduction of a drug into the subarachnoid space of the meninges. A long fine needle with a sharp point is used to pierce the spinal theca and inject the solution into the cerebrospinal fluid.

At the beginning of this century this was a widely-used method of producing analgesia of the lower part of the body but the technique was less frequently employed when it was realised that satisfactory results could be achieved with the new and improved general anaesthetic without the attendant hazards of the spinal method. There were reports of tragic cases of paraplegia, which may have been due to impurities in the solution that were introduced into the cerebrospinal fluid with the injection.

Improvements in pharmaceutical preparations and in aseptic techniques have reduced the risks, and spinal analgesia is now regarded as a very effective alternative to a general anaesthetic.

Epidural analgesia

The drug is injected into the tissues of the epidural space which lies between the dura mater and the layer of periosteum lining the vertebral canal, and the solution infiltrates around the nerve fibres to produce analgesia of the lower half of the body. A spoon-shaped, trocar-pointed needle is directed into the epidural space and, when a continuous analgesia is required, a fine plastic catheter is passed with the needle and left in situ, to allow further doses of the solution to be injected at intervals. Epidural analgesia has proved to be very successful in obstetric practice and is often used for delivery by caesarian section so that the mother is aware of the birth of her baby but does not suffer pain and the baby is not affected by the absorption of drugs.

Caudal block

The epidural injection is given into the caudal canal through a wide bore needle. This procedure produces analgesia of the perineum and is most commonly used for obstetric cases.

Drugs used in local analgesia

Lignocaine   Cinchocaine
Bupivocaine   Amethocaine
Mepivicaine   Procaine
Pilocaine

Complications of local analgesia

1 Toxic reactions due to hypersensitivity to the drug or an overdose.
2 Headaches due to the leakage of cerebrospinal fluid through the puncture hole in the meninges.
3 Accidental injection of the substance into an artery.
4 Infection of the injection site caused by breaks in the aseptic technique.
5 Paraplegia.

General anaesthesia

A general anaesthetic produces a state of unconsciousness and an absence of all sensations. The aim of the anaesthetist is to produce muscle relaxation, analgesia and hypnosis by using either a single anaesthetic agent which produces all these reactions simultaneously, or by balanced anaesthesia, achieved by the administration of several drugs, each having a specific property, which, when used together, will give the desired results with the greatest degree of safety.

Premedication

The premedication that is prescribed by the anaesthetist is usually a combination of drugs which will bring about the following physiological reactions:

1 Sedation.
2 Reduction of bronchial secretions and saliva.
3 Analgesia.
4 The reduction of postanaesthetic vomiting.

These drugs are given orally or by injection at a stated time before the operation. When unavoidable delays and difficulties prevent the pre-medication being administered at the arranged time, the anaesthetist may prefer to give an intravenous injection in the operating department.

Drugs for premedication include:

Morphia
Paperveretum (Omnopon)
Pethidine
Atropine
Hyoscine (Scopolomine)

The induction of general anaesthesia

Intravenous induction of anaesthesia

Anaesthesia is rapidly induced when a solution of an anaesthetic agent is injected directly into a vein on the dorsal aspect of the patient's hand or in the antecubital fossa. This is a safe and convenient means of induction which allows the anaesthetist to inject a known quantity of the drug at a controlled rate.

Drugs commonly used for intravenous induction include:

Thiopentone sodium
Methohexidone sodium
Fentanyl
Ketamine
Diazepam

The induction of anaesthesia by inhalation (Table 9.1)

The open mask method

One of the earliest methods of inducing anaesthesia was by inhaling vapour through a thick pad of gauze laid over a wire frame which covered the patient's nose and mouth. A volatile anaesthetic agent, such as ether or chloroform, was dripped on to the gauze and inhaled by the patient. There was no way of measuring the concentration of the gas which reached the patient and the toxic nature of the substances used in this type of anaesthetic produced distressing postoperative vomiting.

Table 9.1   Summary of the properties of anaesthetic gases and volatile anaesthetic agents

	Properties	
Anaesthetic gases		
Nitrous oxide	Rapid induction and recovery Few postoperative effects	Poor anaesthetic Poor muscle relaxant
Cyclopropane	Good anaesthetic Non-irritant Rapid induction	Respiratory depressant Highly explosive
Volatile anaesthetic agents		
Ether (Diethyl ether)	Good relaxation Minimal cardiovascular depression Deep anaesthetic	Postoperative nausea and vomiting Explosive Highly inflammable, cannot be given when diathermy current is used
Chloroform	Powerful anaesthetic Non-irritant	Highly toxic Postoperative vomiting and nausea
Trichloroethylene (Trilene)	Good analgesic Rapid effect	Poor relaxation Cannot be used in closed circuit
Halothane (Fluothane)	Good anaesthetic Rapid induction and recovery	Poor analgesic Liver toxicity Incomplete muscle relaxation
Methoxyflurane (Penthrane)	Good relaxant and analgesic	Prolonged induction and recovery

Inhalation from an anaesthetic machine

The gases are conducted from an anaesthetic machine, through corrugated tubing to a face mask. Volatile anaesthetic agents may be added to the gaseous mixture and inhaled through the rigid mask.

Apparatus for the inhalation of anaesthetic gases

Anaesthetic machines are used to control the flow of gas to the patient.

Oxygen and nitrous oxide are usually stored in a central supply and carried by pipeline to wall or pendant outlet valves in the anaesthetic room and in the operating theatres.

Cylinders

Gases are also delivered in steel cylinders which are attached to the anaesthetic machine. The nature of the gas in each cylinder is identified by the distinctive colour coding of the painted exterior.

Oxygen	Black with white shoulders
Nitrous oxide	Blue
Carbon dioxide	Grey
Cyclopropane	Orange

Pressure reducing valves

The compressed gases in the cylinders pass through reducing valves to be delivered at a pressure that is suitable for use in the machine.

Flow meter

A rotameter with a spinning bobbin measures the rate at which the gas flows through the machine.

Vapouriser

Vapourisers are containers for volatile anaesthetic agents. The simplest model, used for ether, is comprised of a glass jar to hold the liquid, and a metal U-tube which conducts the gases through the chamber to mix with the vapour from the liquid agent and flow on to the reservoir bag. A more complicated apparatus, used for Halothane, is designed to compensate automatically for variations in the temperature and pressure of the agent and of the ambient atmosphere, to deliver a known concentration of the volatile agent mixed with the nitrous oxide and oxygen.

The reservoir or rebreathe bag

The mixture of gases flows into a rubber bag and the patient inhales from the gases that accumulate in this reservoir. A non-return valve allows the expired gases to be discharged into the atmosphere before the patient inhales more gas from the bag.

Ventilators

Mechanical ventilators are used to assist respiration when the patient is not able to breathe spontaneously. The ventilator consists of bellows enclosed in a sealed chamber and mechanically operated by a pump.

1 Inspiration. The pressure rises within the chamber and forces the bellows to close, and expel the gases contained therein along the tubing into the patients lungs.

2 Expiration. As the pressure in the chamber falls again the bellows expand and are refilled with fresh gases. The expired air from the patients lungs escapes into the atmosphere and the cycle is repeated.

Closed circuit absorption system
When a closed circuit is used for the administration of anaesthetic gases the expired air from the patient passes through a unidirectional valve to a cannister of soda lime which absorbs the carbon dioxide and passes on through the machine, mixing with the gases in the reservoir bag, to be rebreathed. This is an economical method and also avoids pollution of the theatre atmosphere by exhaled anaesthetic agents.

Intubation
Intubation of the trachea is performed during general anaesthesia to maintain an airway when the muscles of respiration are relaxed. An endotracheal tube with an inflatable cuff at the distal end is passed through the vocal cords into the trachea under direct vision from a laryngoscope. The cuff is inflated when the tube is in position to ensure a close fit and prevent regurgitated stomach contents and mucus from entering the trachea and the lungs. Plain or uncuffed tubes are used for intubation by the nasal route during oral and dental surgery.

Muscle relaxant drugs
Muscle relaxant drugs block the transmission of nerve impulses to voluntary muscles to provide the complete relaxation that is required for intubation and surgery. The muscles involved in respiration are paralysed by the action of the relaxants and, therefore, mechanical or hand ventilation must be continued until the effects of the drug have been reversed and spontaneous respiration is established.

Maintenance of anaesthesia
Ventilation with nitrous oxide and oxygen is continued throughout the

operation with the addition of a volatile agent such as halothane or ether. A balanced anaesthetic can be achieved by the inhalation of nitrous oxide and oxygen supplemented with injections of a muscle relaxant and a potent analgesic agent.

Extubation

When the operation is nearly completed the patient is prepared for the return to spontaneous breathing and the reversal of the action of the muscle relaxants. The trachea is aspirated with a suction catheter and a pharyngeal airway is positioned in the mouth. The cuff of the endotracheal tube is deflated and the tube is withdrawn.

Complications during general anaesthesia

During intubation:

1 Respiratory obstruction caused by:
   a Obstruction at the lips.
   b Obstruction by the tongue.
   c Flaccid jaw muscles.
   d Obstruction above the glottis.
   e Kinking of the endotracheal tube.
2 Laryngeal spasm.
3 Injection into an artery instead of a vein.
4 Vomiting and regurgitation.

During the maintenance of anaesthesia

1 Respiratory depression.
2 Changes in heart rate and blood pressure.
3 Hypoxia and carbon dioxide retention.
4 Malignant hyperthermia.
5 Cardiac arrest.

The nurse in the anaesthetic room

The first duty of the nurse in the anaesthetic room is to establish a quiet atmosphere in which the sedated patient can rest undisturbed by noise and clamour. The preparation of a safe environment for the induction of anaesthesia should be completed before the patient arrives in the room.

Preparation of the anaesthetic room

1 Suction apparatus checked and tested ready for use.
2 Piped anaesthetic gas supply and outlets tested according to the routine procedure.
3 Anaesthetic machine and gas cylinders checked and prepared for use.
4 Patient trolley checked to confirm that the tipping mechanism is functioning and the oxygen supply and emergency tray are in position.
5 Intubation trolley prepared with:
   a A selection of endotracheal tubes that have been tested for patency and the cuffs inflated.
   b An inflating syringe.
   c Induction forceps and tube stillette.
   d Two laryngoscopes in working order with secure light bulbs and blades.
   e Swabs, lubricant and bandage or tape.
   f A selection of tube connections.
   g Face mask and pharyngeal airway.
   h Throat spray for topical analgesia.
6 Hypodermic syringes and needles of appropriate sizes and intravenous cannulae.
7 Oscillotonometer or sphygmomanometer ready for use.
8 Intravenous infusion and pressure monitoring equipment available.

Additional special equipment should be available:

Electric thermometers for accurate measurement of peripheral and core temperatures.
Martins pump for rapid blood transfusion.
Oxygen monitoring apparatus.
Insulating blankets.
Paediatric anaesthetic circuits and warming lights for children.
Cardiac monitors.
Cardiac resuscitation trolley.

The reception of the patient

1 Welcome the patient by name and check his identity.
2 Remain with the patient to give reassurance and support.

3 Follow the routine preoperative checking procedure, if this has not already been completed at the transfer area.
4 Check that the patient's head is at the tipping end of the trolley.
5 Arrange for the scrub nurse to see the form signed by the patient giving his consent to the operation.
6 Check and record all drugs required by the anaesthetist.
7 Loosen the clothing around the patient's neck.
8 Apply the blood pressure cuff.
9 Assist in the placing of electrodes and the administration of intravenous infusions.
10 Protect the patient from unnecessary physical and emotional distress or loss of dignity.

Administration of local analgesia

1 Prepare the room and receive the patient as for general anaesthesia.
2 Support the patient in the position required by the anaesthetist.
3 Observe the patient closely and report any physical reactions to the anaesthetist.
4 Warn the patient of impending changes in position or environment and remain close to him throughout the operation.
5 Guard against indiscreet conversation which can be overheard and misinterpreted by the patient.
6 Be prepared to act promptly if complications occur, and assist in the induction of a general anaesthetic if this should be necessary.

Induction by inhalation

During the induction of anaesthesia by inhalation the nurse should stand close to the patient, prepared to give support and ready to assist the anaesthetist if necessary.

Induction by intravenous injection

The nurse's assistance may be required to support the patient's arm while the venepuncture is made and an intravenous cannula is introduced and secured. When the jaw muscles relax the nurse should be prepared to maintain a clear airway by holding the jaw forward. There is a danger that, when the cardiac sphincter is relaxed, regurgitated stomach contents will seep into the oesophagus and enter the trachea to be inhaled into the lungs, with disastrous results. Pressure on the cricoid cartilage during induction will reduce the risk.

The procedure for applying cricoid pressure

1   The table is tilted in a steep head up position.
2   Oxygen is administered by a face mask.
3   The nurse places two fingers of the right hand on one side of the cricoid cartilage and the thumb on the other side, ready to apply pressure when required.
4   When instructed by the anaesthetist, the nurse applies backward pressure on the cricoid cartilage to compress the oesophagus between the cartilage and the body of the vertebra, and prevent seepage into the trachea.
5   The anaesthetist intubates the patient and inflates the cuff of the tube.

Vomiting during induction

It is dangerous to apply cricoid pressure when the patient is vomiting. Using pressure against the positive reaction of vomiting could cause a ruptured oesophagus.

Prompt action is required.

1   Turn the patient on his side.
2   Tilt the trolley or table in the head down position.
3   Provide swabs and suction and assist in clearing the airway.

Precautionary measures are taken when it is suspected that these complications may arise. The stomach is aspirated through a tube, if possible, and the residual gastric contents are neutralised by giving an antacid substance such as magnesium trisilicate or aluminium hydroxide gel.

Intubation

The nurse can assist the anaesthetist by:

1   Passing the equipment as it is required.
    a   Laryngoscope.
    b   Lubricated tube fitted with the appropriate mount.
    c   An empty syringe for inflating the cuff.
    d   A length of tape with which to secure the tube.
2   Positioning the suction apparatus ready for use.
3   Remaining close to the patient, alert, and prepared to respond promptly in an emergency.

4   Remove unwanted covers and blankets before transferring to the operating theatre.

Maintenance of anaesthesia

Assist in the transfer and positioning of the patient on the operating table, being careful to guard the patient's safety and his dignity.

Assist in the administration of intravenous infusions and blood transfusions and checking and recording these procedures.

Extubation

1 Test the suction equipment and attach the laryngeal sucker.
2 Prepare the appropriate size of pharyngeal airway.
3 Assist in the safe transfer of the patient from the operating table to the trolley or the bed.
4 Maintain a clear airway.
5 Oxygenate the patient if necessary.
6 Keep the patient warm.
7 Assist in the transfer to the recovery room.
8 Provide a full verbal report of the patient's response to the anaesthetic and present a written record of the nursing care given during the anaesthetic.
9 Replenish the stock and equipment in the anaesthetic room and leave the room ready for use.
10 Check the stock of drugs in the cupboards and confirm that the records have been completed.

The cleaning and disposal of used equipment

All used anaesthetic equipment should be removed from the operating theatre by the established route for contaminated articles.

Endotracheal tubes, airways, laryngoscope blades, tubing, rebreathe bags and face masks that are to be reused require decontamination and sterilising. Glass phials, syringes and needles must be safely discarded in special, sealed containers.

The surfaces of machines and equipment are cleaned daily with a detergent germicide.

Disposable anaesthetic equipment should be used when it is known that a high risk infection is present and non-disposable items must be processed according to the hospital procedure policy for dealing with contaminated articles from patients with high risk infections.

Further reading

Austin, T R (1977) General Anaesthetic Techniques, NATNews, 14: 29–30

Campbell, D and Spence, A (1980) A Nurse's Guide to Anaesthetics, Resuscitation and Intensive Care, 5th edition, Churchill Livingstone

Jones, B (1980) Pharmacology for Student and Pupil Nurses, Heinemann Medical

Murrin, K R (1978) Local Anaesthesia, NATNews, 15: 10–12

CHAPTER 10

PREPARATION OF THE OPERATING THEATRE FOR SURGERY

Objectives

The nurse will be able to:

1 List the important tasks in the preparation of the theatre for an operation.
2 Describe the correct method of opening sterile packs and packages.
3 Outline the circulating nurse's duties in assisting the scrub nurse in the preparation of sterile trolleys.

Preparation of the operating theatre

Although the operating theatres are thoroughly cleaned at the end of each day, some dust particles will inevitably settle during the time that the theatres are not in use.

At the beginning of the day all the surfaces in the theatre, including the operating lights, table and equipment are cleaned with a disinfectant solution to remove any accumulation of bacteria. The environment is checked to confirm that the ventilation system is functioning and that the recorded temperature and humidity rates are at acceptable levels. (Temperature 22–23°C. Relative humidity 55–60%.)

Before making further preparations it is wise to gather all the available information about the patient, the operation, and the surgeon's methods, by referring to the operating list and the surgeon's preference cards. When the patient has been visited preoperatively in the ward, by a member of the theatre staff, probable nursing problems will have been identified and communicated to the staff who are directly involved in the preparation of the theatre.

Operating theatre equipment

Knowledge of the basic equipment and practise in operating the machines and apparatus is the key to providing a safe environment.

The operating table

The table may be designed with a solid steel mobile base or with a fixed pedestal on to which a transferable top is manoeuvered by a remote control device. The table can be raised, lowered, and tilted, and an extensive range of accessories are produced by the manufacturers to provide support for the patients in all of the positions used in surgery. Some tables are built with an X-ray transluscent top and cassette channels to facilitate radiography during surgery.

The suction apparatus

A suction apparatus complete with laryngeal catheter is provided for the anaesthetist and a separate unit connected to sterile tubing is used by the surgeon for wound suction. The suction is produced by a portable machine with a high vacuum compressor pump or from a central piped system. A pressure gauge indicates the degree of vacuum, which can be controlled as required, from approximately 26 to 5 inches of mercury. The aspirated fluids are collected in a graduated jar which should be autoclavable. The suction tubing, which must be antistatic and of a sufficiently wide bore to prevent blockage, requires constant checking to confirm that it is not accidently kinked or compressed.

The operating lights

These lights are suspended from a complicated ceiling mounting that gives an extensive range of manoeuvrability for focusing the light on the operation site. The light comes from several separate tungsten or halogen lamps set in one large disc holder with the optional addition of a small satellite lamp to provide extra illumination at a different angle.

The operating microscope

Operating microscopes have added a new dimension to surgery, enabling amazingly intricate procedures to be accomplished. Instruction in manipulation, and information on the technical details, should be sought before attempting to prepare or to move these valuable pieces of equipment. The arms of the microscope must be folded in towards the central column, and locked, for even distribution of weight when the unit is to be moved.

The electrosurgery diathermy machine

Electrosurgery or diathermy units that produce an electric current used for sealing severed blood vessels are mounted on mobile trolleys. The relevant cables and accessories are assembled before use and the circuit must be tested according to the manufacturer's instructions.

X-ray machines, monitoring equipment, fibre light sources and other specialised machinery that is requested, is cleaned and brought into the theatre before the operation begins.

Preparing the operating theatre

1 Place the operating table in the correct position and test the mechanism.
2 Collect the table attachments and supports required for positioning the patient.
3 Test the anaesthetic gas pipeline.
4 Connect and test the suction apparatus for the anaesthetist and the suction to be used by the surgeon.
5 Position the intravenous stands, mechanical ventilator and monitoring equipment for the anaesthetist.
6 Connect the diathermy machine and check that the circuits are in working order.
7 Prepare the indifferent electrode, or patient diathermy plate, for application.
8 Adjust the operating lights ready to be focused on the operation site.
9 Check that disposal bags are conveniently positioned.
10 Prepare the scrub-up area with antibacterial lotions and hand-scrubbing brushes.
11 Prepare the swab board and recording form for entering the number of swabs and needles used in the operation and position the receptacles for the collection of used swabs.
12 Prepare for the recording of fluid and blood loss during the operation and check that the weighing scales are available.
13 Provide pathology request forms and specimen containers.

14 Assemble all the packs of linen, instruments and presterilised items that it is anticipated will be required during the operation.
15 Check the location of the emergency resuscitation and defibrillation equipment.

The opening of sterile packages

Preliminary precautions

1 Check the label on the package before opening.
2 Examine the outer covers to check that they are undamaged.
3 Check that the storage time has not expired.
4 Examine the indicator markings to confirm that the package has been exposed to a sterilising process.
5 Never reach over a sterile field or shake the contents of a package on to a sterile surface.

Preparation of the sterile trolleys

1 Position the instrument trolleys and bowl stands ready for draping.
2 Wipe the surfaces with a bactericidal solution or spray.
3 Remove the outer dust cover from the sterile pack before placing it on the trolley.
4 Prepare a sterile trolley in the scrub area for surgical gowns and gloves.

The procedure for opening sterile packs

When the scrub nurse is gowned and gloved, and ready to proceed with the preparation of the sterile trolleys, the outer covers of linen or paper are folded back by the circulating nurse, leaving the sterile inner pack accessible to the scrub nurse.

The circulating nurse handles only the outer surface of the wrapper as she places her hands under the folded edge and draws the cover towards her over the front of the trolley.

The right and left sides are unfolded in the same manner, and finally the fold of the cover on the side where the scrub nurse will stand. By moving around the trolley the circulating nurse avoids reaching over the sterile inner pack.

The procedure for opening sterilising bags sealed with indicator tape

1 Examine the outer wrapping for breaks or damage.
2 Show the label to the scrub nurse.
3 Break the sealing tape.
4 Spread open the gusset on either side of the bag handling only the outer surface of the paper and avoiding contaminating the edges of the opening.
5 Hold the packet horizontally with the opening of the bag facing the scrub nurse, but not extended over the sterile field.
6 Allow the scrub nurse to withdraw the inner packet using sterile forceps.
7 Discard the outer packet.

Opening peelback packages

The circulating nurse grasps the free edges of the packet between her thumbs and peels the two surfaces apart to reveal the sterile contents for the scrub nurse to remove.

Circulating nurse's duties

The circulating nurse stands on the opposite side of the trolley to the scrub nurse, maintaining a safe distance from the sterile field, while she opens sterile packets, pours the lotions and counts the swabs and needles with the scrub nurse.

When the patient has arrived in the anaesthetic room and his identity has been checked, the name of the patient and the operation is posted in a prominent position in the theatre.

The number of swabs and needles in use is recorded on the swab board or chart.

The scrub nurse is shown the signed form giving the patient's consent to the operation and details of any allergies or problems that are recorded in the patient's notes.

Diligent preparation of the operating theatre is conducive to a calm and efficient atmosphere during the operation.

Further reading

Campbell, M and Spence, A (1979) Theatre Routine, 5th edition, Modern Practical Nursing Series, Heinemann Medical

CHAPTER 11

THE CIRCULATING NURSE

Objectives

The nurse will be able to:

1 Enumerate the responsibilities of the circulating nurse.
2 Identify the problems of moving an unconscious patient.
3 List the measures employed to protect patients from injury during positioning for surgery.
4 Explain the importance of measuring blood and fluid loss during an operation.
5 Outline the procedure for the collection and preservation of specimens for investigation.
6 List the duties of the circulating nurse during an operation.

The circulating nurse

One of the most responsible jobs in the operating theatre is that of the circulating nurse. While the scrub nurse is unable to leave the vicinity of the sterile table, the circulating nurse must be prepared to move swiftly to provide extra sterile packs, connect machines, focus lights, manipulate the table and keep accurate records. Operating theatre nurses take pride in achieving high standards of efficiency as circulating nurses and, in some countries, the law requires that the circulating nurse must be a qualified registered nurse.

The responsibilities of the circulating nurse

1 To give direct nursing care to the patient.
2 To protect the patient from harm.
3 To anticipate and supply the needs of the scrub nurse.
4 To conscientiously apply the principles of asepsis and to notify the scrub nurse of suspected breaks in the technique.

The duties of the circulating nurse during the operation

Lifting the patient

Anaesthetised patients must never be moved without the consent of the anaesthetist.

It is important that this manoeuvre is carefully planned and executed because sudden movements and alterations in position can cause circulatory depression and respiratory embarrassment.

Transferring the patient to the operating table

1 Lock the wheels of the patient trolley in position.
2 Adjust the height of the table to correspond to the height of the trolley.
3 Check that the patient's head is safely supported on the stretcher canvas.
4 If the patient is to be lifted, check that the poles are safely slotted into the sleeves of the stretcher canvas.
5 When a roller device is used for transfer to the operating table check that the patient's feet are on the roller before commencing the rotating action.
6 Guard cannulae tubing, cables and drainage bags during the transfer.
7 Supervise and assist in the transfer, to protect the patient from the dangers of sudden movement.
8 Secure the diathermy patient plate electrode.

Positioning the patient for surgery

All the supports and extra accessories should be assembled in readiness for the patient's arrival. The nursing history notes will give information about his general condition and an indication of any special problems that may arise.

The operating table

The mattress must be at least two inches thick and covered with smooth or corrugated antistatic rubber. The ridged surface was originally intended to prevent the patient from slipping, but a smooth rubber is often preferred because it is suspected that the pressure of the ridges on ischaemic tissue causes skin damage.

Special mattresses are used to protect vulnerable patients during long operations. Alternating pressure mattresses, vacuum packs, gamgee and sheepskins are used with success to protect patients from skin damage.

Operating table accessories

Clamps on the side rails hold the supporting rods in position and all the supports are covered with antistatic rubber and thickly padded.

Foam rubber pads

Foam rubber is a versatile substance that can be cut and tailored to individual requirements and is used extensively to protect boney prominences. Pillows, sandbags, polystyrene bean bags and folded towels are utilised for the provision of extra support wherever it is needed.

Positioning the patient on the operating table requires knowledge and skill. Adequate preparation and skilful use of the positioning equipment, and applied knowledge of anatomy and physiology, can be instrumental in preventing complications and injury during surgery. Successful positioning will provide exposure of the operation site for the surgeon, allow access for the anaesthetist and afford maximum safety for the patient without causing him to be unduly exposed.

Physiological problems

An assessment of the general fitness, weight, and skin condition indicates the potential problems of each patient and the precautionary measures required.

Respiratory

Respiratory function can be impaired by restricted chest expansion or obstruction of the airway. When ventilation is interrupted in any way there is danger from carbon dioxide retention and alteration of the arterial blood gas content.

Circulation

Alterations in blood pressure, which occur during anaesthesia, produce circulatory problems for the patient. A lowered blood pressure slows down the return of blood to the heart for reoxygenation, and venous stagnation can predispose to clot formation and deep vein thrombosis.

1 Anti-embolus stockings and alternating pressure leggings are worn as a preventive measure by patients who are at risk.
2 A heel pad or rest, two inches thick, is placed under the achilles tendon to relieve pressure on the calf tissues and vessels of patients in the supine position.
3 A small pillow placed under the right hip relieves pressure on the inferior vena cava caused by the weight of the baby, prior to delivery by caesarian section.

Nerve damage

Nerves are damaged when they are compressed or when they are stretched by hyperextension of a joint. In both instances the area becomes ischaemic, the nerve is damaged and pain and palsy result. The brachial plexus is particularly vulnerable when the patients arm is extended on a board which is abducted at an angle exceeding 90°. Peripheral nerves need protection against compression by careful positioning and securing of the limbs.

Skin injuries

An anaesthetised person must always be moved by lifting or rolling to prevent the damage caused by friction and shearing when the body is dragged into position. Skin and soft tissue require protection from pressure against hard surfaces.

Aims in positioning

1 The achievement of good body alignment.
2 The provision of adequate support where hollows exist between the patient's body and the table surface.
3 Stability and security in the position.
4 Protection of the skin and prominences from injury by pressure and friction.
5 Protection of the patient from the dangers of diathermy burns caused by direct contact of the skin with solid metal.
6 Provision of adequate exposure of the operation site.

Method

1 Straighten the sheets and drapes underneath the patient.
2 Inspect the skin and record any abrasions or redness that requires special attention.
3 Proceed with the positioning when the anaesthetist signifies his approval.

Positions used in surgery

Supine

The patient lies on his back, with his head on a pillow, legs straight and arms resting by his side and supported by an arm retainer. A heel pad or a rolled towel positioned under the heels will elevate the calves and relieve pressure on the blood vessels of the legs.

Additional support provided by:
Anti-embolus stockings.
Alternating pressure leggings.
A padded board to support the patient's arm and to allow access for intravenous injections.
Soft padding for the protection of joints and prominences.

Trendelenberg position

The patient is supine with the knees over the lower break in the table top. When the table is tilted in the head down position, the abdominal viscera falls towards the diaphragm and provides good exposure for surgery involving organs of the abdomen and the pelvic cavity. The foot section of the table is lowered slightly to prevent the patient from slipping. When effective muscle relaxation is achieved it is seldom necessary to tilt the table at an exaggerated angle to obtain reasonable access to the cavity.

Reverse Trendelenberg position

The patient is in the supine position with the table tilted to raise the head and so decrease the blood supply to the neck during thyroid surgery.

Extra supports
Sandbags or pads under the shoulders to extend the neck.
Horseshoe or ring headrest.
Foot rest to prevent slipping on the table.

Lithotomy position

Used for cystoscopic, vaginal and perineal operations.

The patient is placed on the table in the supine position with the buttocks beyond the break in the lower end of the table. The leg stirrups are fixed in position and adjusted at an angle to give maximum exposure without causing undue strain to the leg muscles. The patient's legs are slowly raised and flexed by two people, moving simultaneously, to prevent dislocation of the hip. The feet are placed in the stirrup rests or slings and the foot end of the table is lowered and removed. At the end of the operation the legs are slowly lowered together to rest on the table.

Extra supports

A lumbar pillow.

Padding to prevent contact between the patient's skin and the metal poles.

Foam padding to relieve pressure on the inner surfaces of the legs.

Anti-embolus stockings.

Leg stirrups with padded knee and calf supports which are used during long operations and for patients who are liable to suffer pain and discomfort from over extension of the joints.

Lateral position

During operations on the chest the patient is positioned on the unaffected side with the lower leg flexed and the upper leg straight. The patient is held securely in position by a velcro strap or by wide adhesive plaster attached to the side rails and passed over the patient's hips.

Extra support

A raised arm support for the upper arm to allow adequate chest expansion and a padded board for the lower arm.

A pillow placed between the knees.

Table accessories or sandbags to support the chest and abdomen.

Padding to protect the brachial plexus and the elbow joint.

Inflatable cushions or a raised table rest to elevate the region between the ribs and the pelvis for kidney operations.

Prone position

The patient is turned on to his face with a pillow under his chest, to aid respiration, and another pillow under the ankles. The arms are placed by the patient's side or extended over his head. The head section of the table can be lowered slightly and the patient's head turned to the side and supported on a special rest or pillow.

Extra support and protection
Sandbags and rolled towels placed along the side of the chest.
Pillows or foam pads to place under the abdomen.
Padding to protect the prominences of the iliac crest, shoulders and knees.
Protection for the face and ears.
Head rest.

The jacknife position

A position sometimes used for anal surgery. The patient is placed in the prone position with the hips over the break in the table. The arms are extended sideways and a pillow is positioned under the ankles. The lower end of the table is lowered and the table tilted with the head down.

Extra supports
Armboards to support the extended arms.
Rolled towels or foam pads to protect the brachial plexus.

The sitting position

When sitting is the preferred position for neurosurgery the operating table in general use can be adapted, or a specially-designed chair model may be used. The patient is placed in the supine position and the section supporting the back is raised to an angle of approximately 60° while the whole table is tilted slightly in a head down position. Respiration is unimpaired in this position but there are problems in maintaining a satisfactory circulation and blood pressure.

Extra supports
A head brace or posterior fossa head rest.
Foot rest.
Additional padding for the ischeal tuberosities and the heels.
Pillow on the abdomen on which to rest the patient's hands.

Orthopaedic tables

Specially designed tables are used for some orthopaedic operations. They are equipped with fully adjustable supporting rods to allow access for radiography and surgery and maintain constant traction of the affected limbs during surgery.

The duties of the circulating nurse

The circulating nurse connects the cable from patient plate electrode to the diathermy machine and checks that the catheter and drainage bags are functioning satisfactorily.

When the sterile draping procedure has been completed the furniture and equipment is conveniently positioned around the operating table and the sterile tubing is connected to the suction apparatus. The sterile diathermy cable is attached to the machine, the dials are set, and the foot pedal positioned beside the surgeon's foot. While the operation is in progress the circulating nurse remains at the foot of the table, within sight of the scrub nurse, ready to anticipate and fulfil her needs and to act promptly if an emergency arises.

The measurement of blood and fluid loss

The amount of blood and fluid lost by the patient during surgery is of prime concern to the anaesthetist in calculating the necessity for replacement by intravenous infusion or transfusion. The calculation and accurate recording of fluid loss is particularly important for babies and young children for whom the replacement can be vital.

Swabs   The used swabs are collected and weighed when an estimate of the blood lost is required. The amount is calculated by subtracting the weight of an equivalent number of dry swabs from the gross weight of the soiled ones.

Fluid loss   The amount of body fluid collected in the suction jar is measured by graduations on the side of the container.

Urine drainage   Urine that is draining into a closed container is measured and recorded at regular intervals.

The collection and preservation of specimens

Tissue specimens and biopsies provide vital information for the diagnosis and treatment of the patient and the collection and preservation of these tissues requires careful management.

Preparation

1   Prepare a form bearing the patient's name, hospital number and the relevant details.

2   Prepare a label for the container with the same information.
3   Provide a separate container for each specimen.

Procedure for collecting specimens during operations

1   The specimen is received by the scrub nurse and deposited in a sterile container or it is passed to the circulating nurse with directions for the preservation of the tissue and the labelling of the container.
2   The specimen is deposited in the prepared jar or dish.
3   The nature of the specimen is written on the label which is then fixed to the container.
4   At the end of the operation the form is completed and signed by the doctor.
5   The specimen and label are checked by the scrub nurse and recorded in the nursing notes.
6   All specimens are removed from the theatre before the next operation begins.
7   Details of the specimen are recorded in a special register before it is transferred to the laboratory.

Hospital policy will indicate the procedure for the preservation of samples requiring special containers and those for immediate despatch.

Dissected tissues must never be removed from the theatre or discarded, until the operation is completed and permission has been given for their disposal.

During the operation

The circulating nurse assists the scrub nurse by participating in the counting and recording of swabs, needles and instruments used in the operation. Soiled swabs are collected according to the procedure policy of the hospital.

Messages for members of the surgical team and information concerning changes in procedure and schedules are relayed to the scrub nurse by the circulating nurse.

At the end of the operation

1   Assist in the final count of swabs, needles and instruments.
2   Provide the appropriate wound dressings and skin-cleaning lotion.
3   Disconnect suction tubing and diathermy cables and remove the patient plate electrode.

4   Assist in the safe transfer of the patient to the trolley or the bed.
5   Record intraoperative care in the patient's notes.
6   Dispose of all used items from the theatre.
   a Instruments return to the dirty utility room for cleaning or recycling.
   b Drapes and linen sealed in an appropriate type of bag.
   c Soiled swabs and waste deposited in sealed disposal bags.
7   Confirm that the documentation has been completed.
8   Supervise the cleaning of the operating theatre.

Finally, the theatre is checked to confirm that the used items from the operation have been removed and that the room is cleared and ready for the next operation.

Further reading

Atkinson, L and Kohn, L (1978) Introduction to Operating Room Techniques, McGraw Hill

Nightingale, K M (1976) Out of Sight—Out of Mind, Surgicos Scholar Award

CHAPTER 12

THE SCRUB NURSE

Objectives

The nurse will be able to:

1 Describe the procedure for the surgical hand scrub and the donning of a sterile gown and gloves.
2 Recall the stages in the preparation of sterile instrument trolleys.
3 Outline the procedure for skin preparation and the positioning of sterile drapes.
4 Enumerate the safety precautions to observe in conducting swab, needle and instrument checks.
5 List the scrub nurse's duties and responsibilities during the operation.
6 Describe the immediate postoperative care and the transfer of the patient to the recovery room.

The scrub nurse

The scrub nurse is the member of the surgical team who prepares and preserves a sterile field and keeps account of the swabs, instruments and needles used during the operation. After washing her hands and arms according to the hospital's approved procedure and donning a sterile gown and gloves, the nurse prepares instruments and sutures and passes them to the surgeon as they are required. The scrub nurse has a responsible job requiring anticipation, quick reaction and conscientious observation, as well as a knowledge of anatomy and of operative procedures.

The scrubbing, gowning and gloving procedure

The surgical hand scrub procedure is completed by all the members of the operating team before putting on a sterile gown and gloves. The aim is to reduce the number of transient contaminating bacteria on the skin of the hands and forearms, as a safeguard against dangers from unobserved punctures in the gloves and seepage through the material of the gown sleeves. When an effective antimicrobial soap or detergent is used for the hand scrub, a residue is deposited on the skin surface that will remain active for a limited period when the hands are gloved.

Hexachlorophane and iodine are the chemical agents most often used in these preparations but alternative solutions should be made available for those persons who are allergic to a particular product. Special regimes are recommended by the manufacturers to obtain optimum results from their products but the testing and evaluation of new substances, and the study of research into the subject, is a continuing responsibility of theatre nurses and infection control committees.

The solutions are dispensed from elbow and foot operated containers that require diligent cleaning of tubes and fittings to prevent bacterial accumulation.

When nail brushes are used in the scrubbing procedure these may be the disposable type, backed with a foam pad and impregnated with a suitable disinfecting agent or non-disposable brushes that are resterilised after use and stored in a dispensing container.

Vigorous scrubbing with a hard brush can be painful and cause damage to the skin but light friction or rubbing will produce the desired results. A scrubbing sequence is followed that commences at the fingers and hands and progresses along the forearm to finish above the elbow. The hands are always held above waist level to allow water to drain away from the clean area towards the uncleaned.

Specific instructions to be followed by all members of the scrub team are written in the procedural manual of each operating department.

Preparation for the scrubbing procedure

1 Adjust the headgear to ensure that all the hair is covered and check that the mask fits well and is comfortable and that all jewellery has been removed.
2 The theatre dress or suit may need to be tucked in to prevent loose folds or tapes from brushing against the hands and forearms during

the procedure, and sleeves must be short enough to allow washing above the elbow.

3 Inspect the hands and check that finger-nails are short, clean and free of nail varnish and that there are no open cuts or infected lesions.

The preliminary or social wash

1 Select the water temperature and adjust the speed of flow.
2 Select the antimicrobial soap or detergent agent to be used throughout the procedure.
3 Wash the hands and arms to above the elbows for approximately 2 minutes to remove surface dirt and contamination. Clean the finger-nails, if necessary, with a plastic nail stick.
4 Rinse the soap from the hands and forearms.

The scrubbing procedure

The aim of the scrubbing procedure is twofold. Firstly to separate the bacteria from the skin by friction and secondly to apply an antimicrobial agent that will destroy the bacteria.

This may be achieved by washing the hands and forearms with the agent, or by the use of a brush or sponge, for the prescribed length of time (usually 3–5 minutes). The skin is then rinsed under clear running water.

To complete the process the hands are dried with a sterile towel that is held well away from the body and used to dry one hand and arm, moving in one direction, from hand to elbow and using a circular movement. The used towel is discarded and the process is repeated taking a fresh towel for the second hand.

Gowning

1 Grasp the inner surface of the gown at the neck edge and step back from the trolley. Hold the gown away from the body and let it unfold.
2 Slip the arms into the sleeves of the gown without bringing the hands through the elasticated cuffs and allow the circulating nurse to adjust the gown from behind.

The waist ties of wrap-around gowns that completely cover the wearer's back, can only be tied with assistance from another gowned and gloved person.

Gloving

The open or the closed method of gloving can be used but it is generally accepted that the closed method is safer and less likely to result in contamination of the surface of the gloves by contact with the wearer's skin.

The closed gloving method

The hands are kept within the cuffs of the gown.

1 Grasp the cuff of the right glove with the left hand, keeping it inside the sleeve of the gown, and place the glove on the wrist of the right gown sleeve with the palm facing downwards and the fingers of the glove pointing towards the elbow.
2 Grasp the top of the glove cuff through the sleeve thickness and with the covered left hand, flip the glove cuff over the elasticated cuff so that this is completely covered.
3 Insert the thumb and fingers into the glove while pulling the sleeve into place.
4 Using the gloved hand, place the left glove on the left wrist and proceed as for the right hand.

Open method of gloving

This method is used when changing gloves during the operation when the hands are already through the cuffs of the gown.

1 The hands are brought through the cuffs. Using the right hand, the left glove is picked up by the folded cuff and the hand inserted in the glove.
2 The gloved hand is then slipped under the folded cuff of the right glove and, as the hand slides into the glove, the cuff is stretched over the elasticated cuff of the gown sleeve.
3 The cuff of the left glove is then drawn into position over the left sleeve, using the right hand.

The procedure for assisting in gloving a second person

The gloved person holds the outer side of the glove cuff stretched over the fingers of both hands while the ungloved person plunges a hand into the glove.

When the gloving procedure is completed, the gowned and gloved nurse moves to the laying up area, holding her hands in front of her with the palms together.

The preparation of sterile trolleys and instruments

Careful planning and a methodical approach are needed to adequately prepare the sterile trolleys in the limited time available before the operation begins. The surgeon's preference cards give guidance in the selection of instruments and sutures, but it is logical thinking that aids the scrub nurse in deciding upon the most appropriate order for the preparation and arrangement of the instruments at each operation. Recalling the possible stages of an operation can help in these decisions (Table 12.1).

The area of the room where the scrub nurse stands should be kept clear of equipment and furniture so that she may move freely without fear of contaminating the sterile gown and gloves.

Table 12.1 Types of instruments used at various stages of an operation

Action	Instrument
Incision	Short instruments Cutting—knife, scissors Grasping—artery forceps dissecting forceps Hand retractors
Haemostasis	Coagulating diathermy electrode or forceps
Exposure	Self-retaining retractor
Exploration	Long forceps (7 inches) Artery forceps Dissecting forceps Dissectors and probes Holding forceps
Excision	Clamps Scissors Long handled knife Suction
Anastomosis or repair	Needle holders Dissecting forceps Fine instruments
Closure	Dissecting forceps Tissue holding forceps Scissors

The procedure for the preparation of sterile trolleys

1 The outer covering of sterile packs will have been opened by the circulating nurse in readiness for the scrub nurse to unfold the covers by slipping her hand inside the towels so that her gloved hands do not contact the outer surface of the drapes.

2 For the maintenance of aseptic conditions and for convenience a separate small trolley is used for sutures, swabs and dishes and a large trolley for the instruments.

3 Bowls and receivers are strategically placed utilising all available space but ensuring that no items protrude beyond the edge of the sterile surface.

4 Sufficient drapes are stacked in the order in which they will be required.

5 The mayo tray is draped with a sterile impermeable cover.

6 All the swabs and packs are counted and checked with the circulating nurse.

7 Instruments are counted, inspected and arranged on the sterile surface in the expected order of use. Particular care is required in the placing of cutting instruments. Scissors can be mistaken for artery forceps of the same size and it is unwise to place these instruments side by side.

8 The incision instruments are prepared and positioned ready for immediate use when the operation begins. Knife blades must be guarded and cutting edges protected.

9 A skin cleaning tray or dish is prepared with sponges or swabs mounted on forceps.

10 Sterile diathermy equipment and suction apparatus is assembled.

11 Sutures and ligatures are counted, recorded and left unopened until they are required. A sterile towel can be folded, like a book, with separate layers for opened sutures and ligatures.

12 Extra equipment is tested and prepared.

13 The patient's records showing his name, consent to the operation and any known allergies are witnessed by the scrub nurse.

When the patient is safely positioned, the sterile trolleys are moved into place near the operating table.

Swab, needle and instrument counts

Accounting for the swabs, needles and instruments used in the operation and recording the result is the heavy responsibility of the scrub nurse.

The grave consequences of leaving these foreign bodies in the patient has led to special recommendations issued jointly by the Medical Defence Union and the Royal College of Nursing. Current issues of this booklet should be available to all operating theatre nurses and each hospital should produce a written procedure for the counting of swabs and instruments which it is obligatory for every theatre nurse to read and to observe.

Safety precautions

1 All swabs used in the operating theatre must contain a radio-opaque marker. White swabs are used for surgery and coloured swabs provided for the anaesthetist.
2 Swabs are supplied in various sizes and plys but the fibres from which they are made must comply with standard specifications to ensure consistency in weight and absorbency.
3 Swabs and packs are tied in bundles of five.
4 No swabs should ever be removed from the theatre during an operation.
5 All swabs, needles and instruments must be counted before the operation, before the closure of a cavity and before the closure of the final tissue layer.
6 At least one of the persons involved in the count should be an experienced, trained nurse.
7 The circulating nurse who completes the checks must sign a register that is kept as a permanent record.
8 All slings and tapes opened during the operation must be counted and recorded.

The arrangements for the collection of discarded swabs may vary, but most operating departments use a clear plastic bag or holder for discarded swabs, to eliminate the danger from atmospheric pollution when used swabs hang on a rack for a long period of time. It is essential that the scrub nurse is able to see and account for the used and unused swabs throughout the operation.

Guidelines in handling swabs

1 Check that there are no loose swabs left in the theatre from the previous operation.

2 Packets of swabs in which there is a discrepancy in the number contained in the bundle should be discarded and removed from the theatre.

3 All unmounted swabs are removed from the operating field before a cavity is opened.

4 Radio-opaque swabs must never be used as dressings. They cause confusion in reading postoperative X-rays.

5 A record should be made on the board when a swab is introduced into a cavity during the operation, and when it is removed.

6 When circumstances require the circulating nurse to leave before the completion of the operation, a count should be made with the replacement nurse before the first nurse leaves the theatre.

7 The circulating nurse must see the radio-opaque marker on each of the swabs as they are counted.

8 When there is an interruption during a count, the procedure is restarted.

9 All large swabs with tapes attached should have an artery forcep clipped to the end of the tape when it is introduced into a cavity, unless the surgeon specifically requests otherwise.

10 The surgeon must be informed by the scrub nurse that the swabs, instruments and needles are correct before a cavity is closed. Any discrepancies at the final count must be reported and recorded.

The needle check

Needle checks are made at the same time as the swab check and include all types of needles as well as suture and anastomosis clips. The suture packets containing needles are counted with the circulating nurse and recorded on a board. The empty foil suture packets can be retained to provide an additional check of the number of needles opened and used.

During the operation the scrub nurse takes the used needle from the surgeon before passing a replacement, whenever this is possible.

The discarded and used needles are collected together on the suture trolley. Adhesive pads or containers are the safest means of retaining used needles and displaying them for counting.

Both parts of needles that are accidently broken must be accounted for, and dropped needles should be displayed on the recording board and not removed from the theatre.

Instruments

A similar procedure is used by the scrub nurse before the operation begins and before the closure of the wound. Screw fastenings are tightened, moving parts tested and the instrument examined to determine that it is complete before and after the operation.

Lost items

If the number of swabs, instruments and needles does not tally with the recorded number, the surgeon must be informed and a full search mounted for the missing item. The sterile field is searched by the scrub nurse, and the floor, buckets and furniture by the circulating nurse. All used swabs must be opened, displayed and counted. If the lost item is not located, the patient is X-rayed before leaving the operating theatre and the incident is reported and recorded in the nursing notes and in the operations register.

The skin preparation

When the patient is anaesthetised, the site of the incision and a large surrounding area is made surgically clean before surgery begins.

The skin preparation tray is passed to the surgeon or his assistant who will hand the used tray to the circulating nurse for disposal.

1 The area is examined to ensure that the skin is clean and free from blemishes or infected lesions.
2 The skin is prepared by commencing at the incision site and working towards the periphery until the entire area has been treated by painting the skin with a chemical agent in solution.
3 Potentially dirty areas, such as the umbilicus, should be treated last and the swab or sponge discarded immediately.
4 Spirit-based solutions are used on the skin surfaces and aqueous solutions are used on mucous membrane.
5 The lotion should be evenly distributed to prevent skin damage caused by pooling of the fluid under the patient.

Prepackaged trays complete with sponges and lotion bowls are produced by some manufacturers and the skin preparation is carried out by a gloved assistant massaging the lotion into the patient's skin and leaving the surface thoroughly dried.

The sterile draping procedure

The draping material may be of linen and reprocessed or non-woven and disposable. Disposable drapes are considered to be more costly than linen but there are advantages in knowing that each item is new and unblemished whereas linen threads break and weaken with repeated use.

Permeability of the fabric is an important issue in preventing the migration of bacteria through the drapes to the operation site. When cotton or linen drapes are used there is always a danger of bacterial filtration and a moisture proof layer must be placed next to the patient, underneath the drapes.

Disposable drapes are made of non-woven material that is usually reinforced with a moisture proof substance and repels blood and water.

Guidelines for handling sterile drapes

1   Opened drapes should not be allowed to fall below waist level.
2   Gowned and gloved persons must not reach over an unsterile area.
3   Large sheets should be carried and supported at a level high enough to avoid contamination by contact with unsterile articles and covers.
4   Sterile drapes cannot be repositioned. They must be discarded and replaced.
5   Gloved hands have to be protected by holding them against the inner surface of the drape, within a cuff of the material.
6   Damaged or contaminated drapes must be discarded.

Adhesive plastic skin coverings

These clear plastic sheets offer additional protection against bacterial contamination of the wound by effectively sealing off the area. The drape is applied directly to the skin and firmly fixed by adhesive so that the incision can be made through the plastic covering.

It is recommended that no more than 10% of the total body surface should be covered with this non-porous skin.

The scrub nurse's duties

Thorough and detailed preparation enables the scrub nurse to concentrate on the task of anticipating the surgeon's needs. When the draping has been completed, the sterile trolleys are moved close to the operating table, the light is adjusted, if necessary, and the suction and diathermy tubes and cables are connected to the machines. The incision instruments are handed to the surgeon when the scrub nurse is assured that the preparation is satisfactory and the diathermy dials have been adjusted to the surgeon's requirements.

Experienced and proficient scrub nurses develop a technique by which the instruments are presented with a fluent and flowing motion as one instrument follows another. This skill is only acquired through practice and concentration but it is well worth the effort required to become so closely involved in operations. By following the progress of the operation it is possible to judge the most opportune time for the preparation of sutures and to check swabs so that these and other tasks can be accomplished without delaying the operative procedures. In an emergency or at a critical stage of the proceedings the scrub nurse must give her undivided attention to the operation in order to anticipate and promptly supply the surgeon's needs.

The handing of sterile instruments

All instruments should be handed closed, and screw fittings tightened immediately before passing to the surgeon. The scrub nurse holds the instrument at the joint, or in the middle of the shaft, with the handle pointing towards the surgeon ready for him to grasp. Curved forceps should be held with the tips pointing towards the palm of the nurse's right hand, so that they are directed to the centre of the wound when they are taken by the surgeon.

Knives are grasped halfway along the handle with the cutting edge of the blade facing downwards and covered by the nurse's cupped hand. Throughout the operation the tips of grasping, cutting, and diathermy instruments must be kept clean and free of debris.

At the start of the operation

1 Hand the towel's clips for securing the drapes, if they are required, and secure the diathermy cables and the suction tubing.
2 Pass the incision instruments to the surgeon.
3 Supply the surgeon and his assistants with clean swabs and remove those that have been discarded from the operating field. Pass instruments to the surgeon as they are required.
4 Maintain an uncluttered surface on the mayo tray, with the instruments that are in constant demand neatly arrayed and easily accessible.

5 Prepare sutures as they are required and guard them from loss or damage.
6 Fix used needles and blades to an adhesive or foam pad for disposal.
7 Handle knife blades with care, using a stout needleholder to mount and remove blades and remembering always to turn away from the operating table while performing these tasks.
8 Remove used and unwanted instruments from the operating table and keep them separated from the clean and unused supply.
9 Follow the routine procedure for isolating the wound area during intestinal surgery while the bowel is open.
10 Concentrate on the progress of the operation.

At the end of the operation

1 Before the cavity is closed check all the swabs, needles and instruments and inform the surgeon that the count is correct.
2 Clear the trolley and the mayo tray of unwanted and dirty instruments and place them, opened, in a bowl of cold water.
3 Prepare lotion for cleaning the wound before a dressing is applied.
4 Make a final swab check before the wound is closed.
5 When the dressing has been secured, remove the drapes with gloved hands and deposit in the appropriate receptacle.
6 Remove gown and gloves and dispose of them. Examine the patient's skin for damage or pressure marks and check that the diathermy patient electrode has been removed.
7 Assist in replacing the patient's gown and covers and the transfer from the operating table to the patient trolley.
8 Check that all the instruments are accounted for before they are removed from the theatre.
9 Attend to the recording and documentation of the operation, the specimens and nursing care.
10 Accompany the patient until he is received by the recovery room nurse, to whom a verbal and written report of the patient's condition is given.

Immediate postoperative care

There is sometimes a tendency to hasten the transfer of the patient from the theatre at the end of the operation but this a crucial time when the scrub nurse and the circulating nurse can safeguard the patient and aid his recovery. The first priority is the maintenance of a clear airway and close observation for signs of respiratory embarrassment.

Suction and oxygen equipment should be available and ready for use. It is important to remember that slow redistribution and pooling of blood, following prolonged anaesthesia, causes circulatory problems and hypotension. There may be serious consequences if a patient in this condition is subjected to sudden and erratic movement during the transfer from the operating table.

The restoration of normal circulation is encouraged by keeping the patient warm with adequate coverings. Heated blankets and heat-retaining covers or space blankets are convenient and effective.

The anaesthetist may advocate oxygenation with a venturi mask to help revitalise the tissues before the patient is transported to the recovery room.

Postoperative visit

A postoperative visit is the best source of information for evaluating the effectiveness of intraoperative nursing care and ascertaining whether the goals for the patient were achieved. Alternative arrangements should be made for gathering information concerning the patient's reaction to surgery when a postoperative visit is not possible. In this way the effect of nursing care is constantly reviewed and assessed.

Further reading

Atkinson, L and Kohn, L (1978) Introduction to Operating Room Techniques, 5th edition, McGraw Hill

Medical Defence Union and Royal College of Nursing (1978) Safeguards Against Wrong Operations

Medical Defence Union and Royal College of Nursing (1983) Safeguards Against Failure to Remove Swabs and Instruments from Patients

CHAPTER 13

HAEMOSTASIS IN SURGERY

Objectives

The nurse will be able to:

1 Describe the principle methods used for the control of haemorrhage in surgery.
2 List the types of suture materials available and their properties.
3 Recall the types of suture needles used in surgery.
4 List the safety precautions to observe when electrosurgical diathermy current is used.
5 Describe the procedure for applying a tourniquet to create a bloodless field for surgery.

Haemostasis in surgery

The control of haemorrhage with the minimum of tissue damage is a vital aspect of surgery. The principles employed in haemostasis have been in use since the earliest ages of man but modern technology has introduced sophisticated methods of application, and new materials that have reduced the dangers from tissue destruction, impairment of the blood supply and infected wounds. The principle means of haemostasis used in surgery are as follows:

Pressure

1 Digital pressure is used to control capilliary bleeding at the wound edge.

2   Artery forceps exert pressure on small severed blood vessels and clamp larger vessels before they are divided.
3   Ligatures. Strands of suture material tied around blood vessels to prevent further haemorrhage.
4   Metal clips occlude the lumen of vessels particularly in areas where ligation is difficult to achieve.
5   Sutures. Stitches that approximate wound edges and anastomose tissues also control bleeding.

Heat

1   Hot packs. Large moist hot packs control capilliary haemorrhage over an extensive area.
2   Cautery. A loop of red hot platinum wire for coagulating tissue.
3   Diathermy. A controlled electrosurgical current passed through the patient's body, between two electrodes, to destroy body cells and sear bleeding vessels.

Cold

Cryosurgery. Freezing is used to remove unwanted tissue with controlled haemorrhage.

Chemical reaction

1   Absorbable gelatin, left in situ, assists the clotting process in areas of capilliary bleeding.
2   Oxidised cellulose reacts with the body tissues and swells to form a seal over the area that is bleeding.

Topical thrombin applied to the surface of bleeding tissue as a solution or in powder form.
Bone wax used to plug narrow cavities in bone.
Laser. Intense light beams employed to destroy melanoma and excess tissue without loss of blood.

Indirect means of haemostasis

1   Tourniquets applied to limbs for a limited period of time to present a bloodless field for surgery.
2   Postural haemostasis. Draining the vessels of blood by elevating the limb.
3   Hypotensive anaesthesia. Controlling haemorrhage by the use of anaesthetic agents that block the autonomic ganglia.

Ligatures and sutures

Natural materials of silk, cotton, metals and animal tissues have been used, since prehistoric times, to ligate blood vessels and approximate wound edges. In more recent years synthetic fibres have been developed to produce finer, stronger and less irritant materials which has resulted in presenting a wide choice of sutures for all types of surgery. The strands are supplied in sealed packets that are sterilised commercially by ethylene oxide gas or gamma irradiation.

The classification of sutures

1 Absorbable sutures are broken down in the body tissues and digested by enzyme action within 60 days of insertion.
2 Non-absorbable sutures remain permanently buried in body tissue unaffected by enzyme action.

These sutures are prepared as monofilament or single strands, or multistranded and twisted or braided. Multistranded sutures can be coated, to discourage the capilliary movement of body fluids along the threads, which predisposes to the spread of infection.

Natural absorbable sutures

Catgut is made from beef serosa or the submucosa of sheep's intestine. Single strands are packaged in fluid to keep the material pliable. Catgut is sterilised by gamma rays and cannot be autoclaved.

1 Plain catgut. The untreated strands are rapidly digested by body enzymes. Plain catgut is pale in colour and is most often used for the ligation of superficial vessels and for suturing subcutaneous fat.
2 Chromic catgut. The strands are treated with chromic acid to delay absorption. This catgut is less irritant than the plain variety and is used for structures that heal more slowly.

Despite the introduction of synthetic materials and allegations of variations in tensile strength and absorption rate, catgut continues to be used extensively.

Collagen

Pure collagen fibres from the flexor tendons of beef cattle are prepared as plain or chromisised strands that behave similiarly to catgut, producing minimal tissue reaction.

Fascia Lata

Fascia lata is a living tissue used to strengthen weak fascia in hernia repair.

Handling absorbable sutures

1   The sutures should be used directly from the packet and should not be soaked in water.
2   Store opened sutures between dry towels in a suture book.
3   Exert a gentle pull on the strand to straighten the suture.
4   Refrain from crushing the sutures in artery forceps which weakens the thread.

Synthetic absorbable sutures

Polyglycolic acid is a braided suture that produces low tissue reaction and handles well in use. It is fully absorbed within 60 to 90 days of insertion.

Polyglactin and copolymer are relatively inert and have similar properties to polyglycolic acid.

Non-absorbable sutures

Non-absorbable sutures are used for permanent suturing and for skin stitches.

Silk sutures are made of raw silk from the silkworm which is braided, and may be coated to render the threads serum proof and resistant to capilliary action. Silk is used dry because it loses strength when it is moist.

Cotton gains strength when wet and should be moistened before use. The fibres are twisted and the suture handles well, but lacks strength.

Linen is similar to cotton and is used in gastrointestinal surgery.

Synthetic materials

Polyamides. Nylon is made as a mono- or multifilament suture that is strong and non-irritant. The threads are springy and knots tend to slip unless several extra throws are made. Monofilament nylon is used for tension sutures in abdominal wounds.

Polyester. This is a strong, inert, braided suture that is coated with teflon or silicone when it is used for cardiovascular surgery to allow the thread to pass smoothly through the tissues. The sutures can be used wet or dry and can be autoclaved up to three times.

Polyethylene. Monofilament fibres that are strong and pliable are particularly suitable for hernial and fascial repair.

Polypropylene. This material can be used in the presence of infection and is strong and inert. Polypropylene is used for tension sutures and for fascial repair and can be autoclaved two or three times.

Metallic sutures

Stainless steel makes a strong, inert and flexible suture but requires careful handling to prevent it from becoming twisted and breaking.

Tantalum is another inert metal that can be produced as a very fine suture or as a mesh for hernia repair.

Monofilament silver wire is similar to steel and can be used for supporting a complete rectal prolapse.

Suture sizes

The size of the suture is given on the outside of the packet, together with other relevant information and the code number provided by the manufacturer for identification and for re-ordering of stock.

The size of the suture may be given in both metric and BPC numbering.

The metric sizing is the more accurate as it is related to the diameter of the suture. The size is calculated by multiplying the diameter by 10 (e.g. 0.40 mm = metric size 4).

In the BPC system the thicker sutures are identified by single numbers before a decimal point. The higher numbers denote thicker sutures (e.g. 2 is thicker than 1).

Noughts added after the decimal point indicate the finer threads (e.g. 000, written as 3/0, is finer than 00, or 2/0).

Metal clips

Metal clips or staples of inert metal are used for the closure of skin and fascia, to occlude blood vessels and for anastomosis.

Skin closure

Metal clips have been used for skin closure for many years but recently new designs, presented in presterilised cartridges with disposable applicators, have made the use of clips for the approximation of skin edges safer, simpler, and more efficient.

Prepackaged arterial clips are supplied in various lengths and sizes for the secure and accurate occlusion of blood vessels.

Staples. A cartridge of stainless steel clips is loaded into a stapling gun for speedy and accurate closure of the fascia layer. Anastomosis of the gastrointestinal tract can be made with staples loaded into an anastomosis stapler from which they are ejected to produce a satisfactory union.

Adhesive skin closure strips are used in addition to, or instead of, skin sutures.

Packaging

Sterile suture material and clips are delivered in sealed packets. Precise instructions for opening the packets and handling the contents are supplied by the manufacturers.

Needles

There are a number of factors for the surgeon to consider in the choice of surgical needles for each stage of the operation (Figure 13.1).

Size

The length of the shaft is measured in millimetres and the diameter varies from fine gauge for microsurgery to heavy gauge for tough structures.

Shape

Straight needles. Used mainly for skin suturing.

Curved needles. Three-eighths of a circle used for skin suturing and tension sutures.

Half circle needles mounted on a needleholder for suturing in confined spaces.

Five-eighths of a circle needles are large and held in the hand.

J-shaped needles are used for suturing in areas where access is difficult.

Types of needle

Although there are basically two types of needle, cutting and round bodied, numerous variations in the shape of the point, and the shape and gauge of the shaft, provide a wide range from which to select a suitable needle for each suture.

Symbols on the packet illustrate the shape of the point and of the shaft of the needle.

1   Round-bodied needles have a sharp taper point for passing through delicate tissues.

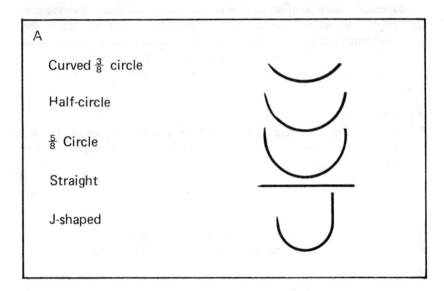

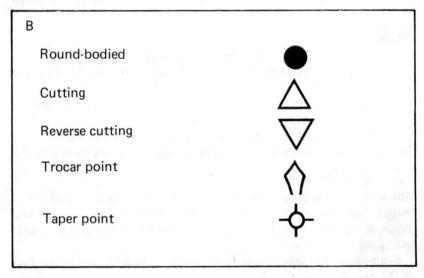

Figure 13.1   a. Shapes of surgical needles. b. Symbols that depict the shapes of surgical needle points.

2   Cutting needles have triangular points and an oval shaft.
3   Taper cut needles have a short fine triangular point.
4   Trocar point needles are heavy gauge for tough tissue.

The eye of the needle

Eyed needles have a large round or oval eye to allow the material to pass through without damage to delicate threads. These needles can be rethreaded and reused throughout the operation. Eyeless or atraumatic needles have the suture welded into the shaft of the needle. There is less trauma from drawing the single thread through the tissue than with a threaded, eyed needle, and as the needles are not reusable, each one is new and sharp.

Atraumatic or eyeless needles are produced in numerous permutations of suture materials and needles to provide an ever increasing range for use in all types of surgery.

Mounting needles on the needleholder

1   Select the appropriate needle and holder. Choose a needleholder with fine tips for fine gauge needles and instruments of heavier metal for the thicker needles.
2   Clamp the shaft of the needle in the tips of the needleholder at about one quarter of the distance from the point to the eye of the needle.
3   Thread the suture through the eye and draw the short end through, for at least three inches.
4   Pass the needleholder to the surgeon with the tip of the needle pointing to his left and hold the free end of the suture to protect it from being contaminated. (The needle is mounted with the tip pointed in the opposite direction for left-handed surgeons.)
5   Mount atraumatic needles in the same manner, clamping the needle at about one quarter of the distance from the welded end to the point.

Stitches used in surgery

Transfixion stitch. A length of suture material is threaded on a needle and passed through the structure before the thread is tied, to prevent the ligature from slipping.

Purse string suture. Running stitches are placed in a circle around an opening and drawn tightly together to prevent seepage.

Stay sutures. A length of suture thread is stitched through the wall of a structure and anchored to elevate the tissues.

Tension sutures

Wounds that are liable to be subjected to extra stress or delayed healing are strengthened by deep tension sutures.

Heavy non-absorbable sutures are mounted on long curved needles and passed through the layers of skin, fascia, and sometimes peritoneum, to draw the wound edges together with interrupted stitches. The underlying skin is protected by small sleeves of plastic tubing or by a rolled gauze strip over which the knot is tied.

Continuous suturing is used to close the lining of a cavity or for anastomosis.

Interrupted sutures are single stitches for strengthening.

Electrosurgical diathermy

Diathermy is the name used for the method of controlling haemorrhage by passing a high frequency electrosurgical current through the patient's body. Heat is produced where the body cells resist the current and the tissues are destroyed or coagulated.

Unipolar diathermy

The current is produced by the machine and conducted to a small active electrode which is brought into contact with the tissues. The current is conducted, by electrolytes and muscle, through the patient's body, to the patient plate, which is a large dispersive or indifferent electrode, and thence to earth, through the machine. The machine is activated by a foot switch and controlled by dials on the machine.

Bipolar coagulation

Coagulation occurs when the current is passed between the tips of forceps which form electrodes of equal size and is not conducted through the patient's body. A patient plate is therefore not required. The low powered current that is transmitted by this circuit can be used for coagulation of fine structures.

The uses of diathermy in surgery

1 Coagulation. Sealing severed blood vessels.
2 Fulguration. The tissues are charred and a scab is formed. The method is employed for the removal of papillomata of bladder.
3 Cutting. The division of tissues. Used for the excision of carcinoma

because the searing of tissues prevents the spillage of malignant cells.
4 Desiccation or blending. The cutting current is combined with coagulation to control haemorrhage.

Active electrodes for unipolar diathermy

The active electrodes and the connecting cables are sterilised and require the same attention as other instruments used at the operation. Insulated instruments and cables should be examined to ensure that the covering is intact, and the tips of forceps need constant cleaning to keep them free of debris. The diathermy instruments must be housed in an insulated holder when not in use during the operation, to prevent accidental burns from unprotected active electrodes.

Types of active electrodes

1 Spatula or heavy point for coagulation.
2 Fine points for cutting.
3 Ball and button applicators for searing areas of vascular tissue (e.g. the liver).
4 Insulated instruments (e.g. forceps and scissors).
5 Electrodes to pass through endoscopic instruments.

The indifferent electrode or patient plate

The indifferent electrode is not sterile and is applied before the sterile drapes are positioned.

Types of indifferent electrode

When lead patient plates are used special attention is required to ensure that the entire plate and attachment is covered by 16 thicknesses of cotton material soaked in isotonic saline solution. If the material dries out the plate ceases to provide conductivity and the patient may suffer a severe burn.

Flexible metal and foil electrodes

These electrodes are either disposable, for once only use, or are intended for limited reuse before disposal. Conductive gel or special adhesive is supplied by the manufacturers to improve the contact between the patient's skin and the plate. Babies can be wrapped in a sheet of aluminium foil during surgery to assist in retaining body heat, as well as providing an effective indifferent electrode.

The positioning of the indifferent electrode

The positioning of the indifferent electrode requires careful consideration to ensure that good contact is maintained throughout the operation. The plate should be positioned as near as possible to the operation site, but not located over an implanted prosthesis, and away from electrocardiograph electrodes. Fat is a poor conductor of electricity, skin becomes ischaemic during long operations and boney and hairy areas do not provide good contact. A muscular area, like the thigh, which has a good blood supply, is therefore selected for the application of the plate.

Safeguards in the use of diathermy equipment

1 Test all circuits of the machine according to the maker's instructions.
2 Discard broken cables and faulty accessories.
3 Check that the patient plate is free from wrinkles and is intact.
4 Apply the recommended gel or adhesive as directed.
5 Fix the plate firmly in position.
6 Check that the cable connections are secure.
7 Prepare the machine with the dials set at 0 until the cables are connected. Audibly check the dial settings when alterations are made.

Diathermy burns

Diathermy burns are liable to occur when the patient's skin is in direct contact with solid metal. The current is diverted from the route between the active and the indifferent electrodes and is attracted to the metal, causing tissue destruction at the point of contact, which is where the current leaves the body. Faulty connections between the patient plate and the cable, inadequate contact between the patient and the plate, and failure to apply a patient plate, can all result in painful and serious burns.

Although modern machines are equipped with fail-safe devices and warning lights, accidents can still occur through negligence and failure to follow instructions and observe safety precautions.

Cautery

When cautery is used a loop of platinum wire is made red hot by low voltage electric current from a battery or a transformer. The heated wire causes coagulation of the tissues and was formerly used extensively in ear, nose and throat surgery but bipolar diathermy, cryo, and laser beams are beginning to replace cautery in modern surgery.

Cryosurgery

The value of intense cold in producing haemostasis and analgesia was recognised by the ancient Egyptians. The same principle is used in modern surgery for the destruction of diseased tissue without pain or bleeding. Controlled bleeding is produced by applying a probe that is reduced to a temperature of minus 20 degrees ($-20°C$) to minus 150 degrees ($-150°C$) by contact with nitrous oxide gas or liquid nitrogen. The tissue clings to the tip of the probe and is released by rewarming the probe.

The use of cryosurgery has extended to all types of surgery as more efficient applicators and machines are developed.

The manufacturer's instructions must be followed for testing, sterilising and maintenance of each unit.

Laser beams

A 'light amplification by stimulated emission of radiation' or laser, produces an intensely bright beam of light that prevents bleeding as it cuts through tissue. The light is contained in a spreading beam that can be directed on to a specific point to remove tissue with no loss of blood. Various sources of laser beams are used in surgery, notably ruby, argon and carbon dioxide.

Because the high intensity beams cause damage when they are reflected by highly polished surfaces, windows must be blacked out and all personnel in the theatre while the laser is in use are provided with protective goggles and asked to remove watches and jewellery. The instruments are made with matt surfaces and a vacuum suction is incorporated in the equipment to prevent the inhalation of injurious fumes.

Tourniquets

Inflatable cuffs are used as tourniquets to stop the flow of blood to an operation site on a limb. The pneumatic cuff can be inflated with air by a hand pump or automatically filled with a noninflammable gas to raise the pressure. When a bloodless field is needed for surgery, the limb is drained before the cuff is inflated, by elevating the part to allow the blood to drain from the vessels. The peripheral vessels are emptied by compression with a rubber Esmarchs bandage tightly wound round the drained limb from the fingers or toes to the level at which the cuff has been applied. There are three sizes of cuff available, a large size for the lower limb and a medium for the upper limbs of adults, and a small cuff for children. When the preparations for surgery have been completed, the pressure in the cuff is raised to the figure directed by the surgeon and the bandage is removed.

Because there is a limit to the length of time that tissues can remain ischaemic, the nurse records the time at which the pressure was raised and reminds the surgeon at regular intervals of the time that has elapsed since the cuff was inflated.

The tourniquet is never released until instructions for deflation are given by the surgeon, and then the patient is only moved very gently and is closely observed for signs of circulatory disturbance. A final check is made before the patient leaves the operating theatre to confirm that the tourniquet has been removed and that the circulation is satisfactory.

Further reading

Aries, J M (1978) Haemostasis in Surgery, NATNews, 15: 22–32

Codes of Practice (1983) National Association of Theatre Nurses

CHAPTER 14

SURGICAL INSTRUMENTS AND WOUND DRAINAGE

Objectives

The nurse will be able to:

1 Classify instruments according to the function that they fulfil in surgery.
2 List the information that is required by the scrub nurse in order to select appropriate instruments for each operation.
3 Describe the factors to consider in the effective care and cleaning of surgical instruments.
4 Enumerate the types of wound drainage used in surgery.

Surgical instruments

The identification of surgical instruments and the selection of those that are most suitable for each operation is a special responsibility of the scrub nurse that requires perseverance to memorise the names and uses of each item, and a logical approach to select the particular instruments required for each individual operation. The choice of instruments is principally influenced by the type of operation to be performed, the patient's size and the surgeon's own preferences.

The classification of surgical operations

Operations can most usefully be categorised according to the reasons for surgery.

1   Excision of cysts and tumours, e.g. prostatectomy.
2   Removal of diseased or infected organs, e.g. appendicectomy.
3   Reconstruction, replacement and repair, e.g. hernia repair, total hip replacement.
4   Transplantation and grafting, e.g. kidney transplant, coronary artery graft.
5   Exploration and investigation, e.g. biopsy, endoscopy.
6   Drainage, e.g. colostomy, cystostomy.

Instruments

Materials and design

Special instruments are made for all the various types of operations. They are manufactured with care and precision to fulfil a particular function and each one must conform to standard specifications.

A stainless steel alloy is the most widely used metal because it combines qualities of durability and hardness with resistance to corrosion and rust. Surfaces are usually shining and bright except when the instruments are intended for use in microsurgery or when reflected light could be hazardous to the surgeon.

Tungsten carbide is often incorporated to reinforce the jaws of needleholders so that, even with repeated use, the hard surface will retain the ability to grip the needle firmly.

Instruments that are designed for use with electrosurgical diathermy current are insulated by a nonconductive material encasing all of the instrument except the working tips and the cable attachment.

Clamping and grasping instruments have jaws on which fine parallel teeth on one blade fit accurately into those on the opposite surface. Some forceps that are used for delicate arterial surgery are especially designed with very small interlocking serrations and a central groove that ensures that the blood vessels are occluded with minimal trauma to the delicate linings of these structures.

Box type joints that have two parts slotted together during the forging process, when the metal is red-hot and malleable, are stronger and longer lasting than joints made by securing two blades together with a screw.

Names of instruments

1   Use. Instruments are named according to the use for which they are intended, e.g. gall bladder clamp, tissue holding forceps.

2 Designer. The name of the designer is added to identify the many patterns and modifications of each type of instrument, e.g. Moynihan gall bladder clamp, Lane's tissue holding forceps.
3 Size. Most instruments are made in a variety of sizes, diameters and lengths and it is necessary to know the size of each one, e.g. 7 inch Lane's tissue holding forceps.

The classification of instruments

Surgical instruments can be grouped according to the purpose for which they are designed.

1 Cutting and dissection, e.g. knives, scissors and dissectors.
2 Grasping and holding, e.g. dissecting forceps, tissue holding forceps, bone holders.
3 Clamping, e.g. artery forceps, intestinal clamps, arterial clamps.
4 Exposing, e.g. retractors, speculae.
5 Investigating, e.g. probes, endoscopic instruments.
6 Suturing, e.g. needleholders, clip applicators.

Basic instrument sets

Sets of instruments are assembled, consisting of a sufficient number of instruments from each group to provide instrumentation for basic surgical procedures.

Sterilised basic sets are prepared and kept in readiness for emergencies.

The selection of instruments

Information required:

1 The age, sex and size of the patient. Smaller instruments will be required for a child or a small female than for a male adult patient.
2 The operative procedure. A knowledge of the stages of the operation will indicate the type of instruments that will be needed (Table 14.1).
3 The surgeon's preference for using a special pattern of instrument, e.g. needleholder.

This information is utilised to select extra instruments to add to the basic set (Table 14.2).

In operating departments where the instruments are prepared in a sterilising unit it is essential that an accurate description of the contents

Table 14.1   The use of surgical instruments in operations

Stage of operation	Instrument	Function
Incision	Knife	Cutting
Haemostasis	Artery forceps	Clamping
Isolation	Tissue-holding forceps	Grasping
Exposure	Retractor	Retraction of tissues
Exploration	Probe	Investigation
Excision	Scissors	Cutting
Drainage	Suction	Aspiration
Closure	Needleholder	Suturing

Table 14.2   Basic instrument set

Dissecting forceps	Toothed 5 inch Nontoothed 5 and 7 inch
Knife handles	For small and large blades
Scissors	Straight 5 inch Curved 5 inch Fine dissecting Round-ended (assistants)
Artery forceps	Curved 5 inch Straight 7 inch Curved 7 inch
Tissue holding forceps	Heavy (e.g. Lanes) Light (e.g. Allis)
Needleholders	5 inch 7 inch
Retractors	Short blade hand retractors Self-retaining retractors
Suction nozzle and tubing	
Diathermy	Cable attachment, instruments and quiver
Sponge holding forceps	

is attached to each package, to avoid confusion and frustration in selecting the correct instruments for each operation.

Power driven instruments

Electrically or pneumatically driven drills and saws operate with speed and precision that causes less trauma and pain than hand operated instruments.

The interchangeable attachments must be firmly secured and the instrument tested immediately before use. The handpiece must not be immersed in water, but can be gas or steam sterilized with the component parts of the instrument.

Endoscopic instruments

1 Give the surgeon an illuminated view of the inner surface of body structures.
2 Provide an opportunity to perform minor surgical procedures without making an incision.
3 Present the means of procuring tissue biopsies for investigation.

Each instrument should be stored and sterilised complete with all of the interchangeable parts and attachments.

A procedure for the cleaning of flexible fibreoptic endoscopes is prepared by each hospital, and specially designed tables are available incorporating cleaning equipment and a tray with separate compartments to accommodate these valuable instruments and accessories.

Prosthesis and implants

Prosthetic devices for the replacement of body structures bring increased mobility, freedom from pain and a longer expectancy of life to the patient. The range and competency of these implants has rapidly developed with the discovery of new materials and techniques.

Metal

Components for the replacement of joints and the strengthening of bones are usually made of metal alloys that remain inert and resist corrosion when they are surrounded by body tissues. Because these metal alloys are not always compatible, the implants made of one metal should be secured with fixing devices made of the same type of metal, e.g. stainless steel bone plates secured with stainless steel screws.

Damage to the surface can cause bone erosion when the prosthesis is implanted in the body.

Prosthesis can be protected by:

1 Encasing the prosthesis in a protective covering of soft material.
2 Sterilising in special containers.
3 Careful handling and protecting from contact with heavy metal objects.

Silicone

Silicone rubber is a soft pliable material that is ideal for the reconstruction of tendons and small bones and for achieving cosmetic effects with breast implants.

This material requires cleaning before sterilisation to remove the dust and oils that cling to the surface and could produce a tissue reaction.

Synthetic materials are used in various and ingenious ways to replace blood vessels, repair muscle defects and assist the functioning of vital organs. The manufacturers supply detailed instructions for the preparation and sterilisation of their products which must be followed, if satisfactory results are to be achieved.

The care of surgical instruments

Instruments and equipment must always be examined and tested before and after use. The patient's life could be endangered if an instrument that is not functioning properly is given to the surgeon during surgery.

The inspection of instruments

1 Check that the instrument is complete and all of the parts are in working order.
2 Tighten screw fittings.
3 Test the joints of hinged instruments to ensure that they move smoothly.
4 Ensure that the ratchets grip firmly.
5 Confirm that the tips of forceps are in alignment.
6 Test the sharp edges of cutting instruments and replace those that are chipped or blunt.
7 Examine insulated instruments for cracks and damage to the covering.
8 Look through telescopes to check that there are no spots or marks on the lenses.
9 Check that the central channels of cannulated instruments are patent.

Damage to instruments

The most common causes of damage to instruments are:

1 Careless handling. Fine instruments should be handled individually and separated from heavy metal objects.
2 Misuse. The use of instruments for purposes other than those for which they were designed.
3 Ineffective cleaning. Dirt and debris lodged in the joints of forceps causes stiffness and corrosion.
4 Neglecting to protect the tips of fine instruments.
5 Allowing the sharp edges of cutting instruments to knock against metal objects.
6 The use of oil lubrication that leaves a residue which is difficult to remove and forms a barrier to effective sterilisation.
7 The use of abrasives that damage the metal surface.
8 Unsuitable detergent solutions and failure to rinse instruments thoroughly after washing.
9 Neglecting to dry instruments after use, to remove dust particles from the surface and moisture from the joints.
10 Failure to follow the manufacturer's instructions that are supplied with special instruments and new equipment.

Cleaning used instruments

1 Immerse in clear cold water as soon as possible after use.
2 Examine and check that all the parts are intact.
3 Disassemble all the components and open jointed instruments.
4 Thoroughly clean the central channels.
5 Wash in detergent solution.
6 Rinse in clear water.
7 Dry and reassemble.
8 If lubrication is needed use a water-soluble solution.

The washing process

The washing process may have to be completed by hand when there are no other facilities but mechanical washing machines, when they are available, are efficient and labour-saving.

Washing by hand Wash instruments in a suitable detergent solution using a soft brush to clean the teeth and box joints. Rinse thoroughly and dry all the parts well.

clean the teeth and box joints. Rinse thoroughly and dry all the parts well.

Mechanical washing machine   Many of the machines in use have an action similar to that of a dish washer. During an automatically timed cycle, water is sprayed from revolving jets, detergent solution washes the instruments and there is a final clear rinse.

Washer–steriliser machines   Used instruments are loaded directly into these fully automatic machines after the operation. During the cycle, the instruments are thoroughly washed with detergent solution, rinsed and sterilised.

Ultrasonic washer   High frequency sound waves are passed through a tank of detergent water causing vibrations that dislodge small impacted particles of dirt without damage to the metal. This method is particularly effective in cleaning delicate instruments but it is not suitable for articles made of rubber, soft plastics or wood, which absorb ultrasonic waves.

The preparation of instruments for sterilisation

1   All articles to be sterilised must be thoroughly cleaned and inspected.
2   Hinged instruments should be opened or locked on the first ratchet only, to allow heat and steam to penetrate to all surfaces.
3   Basic instrument sets are arranged on trays and can be wrapped in drapes ready for use.
4   Single instruments are packed in two layers of sterilising paper.
5   Packages must be labelled with an exact description of the contents and an indication of the processing date.

Wound drainage

The purpose of wound drainage is the removal of air or fluid from a cavity by the formation of a channel or route to a suitable site on the body surface where the fluid is allowed to soak into a dressing or is directed into a closed container by connecting tubing.

The closed system is generally preferred as it is a safeguard against the entry of bacteria into the cavity and provides a means of measuring the quantity of drainage in a graduated container.

Most wound drains are anchored to the skin by a suture and a safety pin fastened across the lumen of the tube, as a precaution against displacement of the drain.

Wound drains are packaged and sterilised individually so that a large selection of types and sizes is available for immediate use.

The materials used for drains must be pliable, non-irritant and soft. Red rubber causes an irritant reaction but latex and silicone rubber, and some plastics, give satisfactory results.

Types of drains

Tube drains and catheters allow a free flow of fluid.

Corrugated drains shed the fluid away from the cavity and on to the surface to drain into a dressing.

Penrose drains are made of fine latex rubber with a gauze strip passed through the lumen to act as a wick.

Chest drains: tubes are inserted in the pleural cavity to drain fluid or air into an underwater seal bottle that is positioned at a much lower level than the patient's chest to encourage drainage by gravity into a fluid trap that prevents an influx of air from entering the chest cavity.

Closed vacuum suction

Fine plastic or silicone tubes with multiple perforations at the distal end, are inserted with a needle introducer that guides the tube through the tissues and to the body surface by piercing the skin. The tube is connected to tubing that is attached to a bottle in which a vacuum has been created.

These fine drains do not usually need to be secured with a stitch, and the gentle withdrawal of exudate and blood from the wound tissues reduces the necessity for pressure bandaging that predisposes to ischaemia and necrosis.

Further reading

Brigden, R (1980) Operating Theatre Techniques, Churchill Livingstone

Dixon, E (1982) Theatre Technique, Baillière Tindall

Westaby, S (1982) Wound Care No 7, Wound Drainage, Nursing Times, 78: centre pages

CHAPTER 15

POSTANAESTHESIA AND RECOVERY ROOM NURSING

Objectives

The nurse will be able to:

1 List the essential equipment for a recovery room.
2 Describe the observations and nursing care of a patient on admission to the recovery room.
3 Name the complications that may occur during the postanaesthetic period.
4 Relate the procedure in the event of a cardiac arrest.
5 List the precautions for safety in the recovery room.

Postanaesthesia and recovery room nursing

Recovery rooms are situated near to the operating theatre, and easily accessible for the surgeons and anaesthetists, with a convenient exit to the perimeter corridor and the return route to the wards. The room is divided into bays, each fully equipped with suction, oxygen, and the necessary supplies for observation and the nursing care of a patient immediately after surgery. The patients, who are accommodated on trolleys, or are transferred to a bed, are cared for by staff who are specialists in postanaesthetic nursing and who strive to provide a quiet and calm atmosphere for the return to consciousness after the operation.

General equipment in the recovery room

A cardiac arrest and resuscitation trolley conveniently positioned and prepared for immediate use.
Cardiac monitors and electrodes.
Rectal and oesophageal thermometers.
Rewarming blankets and fans.
Supplies of fresh linen.
A communication and alarm system.

Equipment for individual bays

The piped gases and suction outlets are either suspended from a ceiling beam or fixed at a convenient height on the wall.
Suction apparatus and catheters.
Oxygen supply with flowmeter and oxygen masks.
Sphygmomanometer.
Thermometers.
Intravenous infusion sets and cannulae.
Dressings and tissues.
Recording chart.
Disposal bins.

Admission to the recovery room

The nurses who care for the patient during the postoperative period provide nursing care and observe each individual patient's response to surgery and anaesthesia. They are a vital link in the continuation of care planned for the patient.

Knowledge of the previous history and treatment are valuable guides in assessing the present reactions, and in recording observations during the recovery period. Every patient needs the individual attention of a nurse to observe, assess and respond promptly to changes in his condition at this critical time.

The procedure

1 The identity of the patient is checked with the operating theatre nurse who gives a verbal account of the operation performed and the condition of the patient on leaving the operating theatre.
2 The nursing and medical notes are handed to the recovery room nurse, and relevant instructions explained.
3 When the anaesthetist has accompanied the patient, he is able to

supply the recovery room nurse with details of the anaesthetic agents used and to discuss instructions for future medication.

4 The patient is observed to confirm that respiratory function is adequate; skin colour, pulse rate and temperature are satisfactory.

5 The vital signs are monitored and recorded at regular intervals:
   a Blood pressure.
   b Temperature.
   c Pulse rate.
   d Respiratory rate and volume.

6 Blood transfusions and intravenous infusions are checked and continued according to the instructions given.

7 Wound dressings, drains and catheters are checked for haemorrhage and excessive drainage. Fluid and urine output is recorded.

8 As the patient regains consciousness, the degree of pain he is experiencing is assessed, and pain relief is administered as directed.

9 Reassurance and comfort are given to the patient as he emerges from anaesthesia and regains full consciousness.

10 Renewal of soiled linen, cleansing of the face and hands and repositioning will add to the patient's bodily comfort.

Hearing is one of the first senses to be recovered after anaesthesia. Nurses are warned to refrain from discussing the patient's condition near the bedside when they appear to be unconscious. The conversation may be recalled by the patient and cause deep distress and anxiety.

The recovery room nurse needs information about the patient to help in identifying possible problems and planning the nursing care in the postoperative period. The nursing history, care plans and notes are useful sources of information, but talking with the patient, during a personal or group interview, often reveals signs of anxiety and tension, previously unnoticed, that can be alleviated by describing the recovery room and giving assurance that the patient will not be left alone.

The most satisfactory arrangement is for the patient to be visited before operation, met at the reception area, accompanied to the anaesthetic room and nursed postoperatively by the same nurse. Busy operating schedules do not often permit this ideal arrangement, but every theatre nurse should, at some time, care for a patient through all the stages of the perioperative period, from the preoperative visit to the return to the ward and the evaluation. This is an experience that is invaluable to the nurse in developing an understanding of the physical effects of surgery and the emotional stress involved.

Complications during the postoperative period

Respiratory complications

To relieve an obstructed airway:

1 Pull the jaw forwards and upwards to prevent the tongue from blocking the airway.
2 Clear the nasopharynx of accumulated mucus by using suction.
3 When the airway is patent, ventilate the patient with oxygen.

Respiratory insufficiency

When the airway has been cleared but the patient's colour remains poor and respirations are shallow and slow, oxygen and air, administered by an Ambu bag, may be effective in aiding respiration until the cause has been diagnosed and treated.

Circulatory problems

1 Tachycardia can be an indication of haemorrhage.
2 Hypotension. Nurse the patient in a supine or lateral position until he is fully recovered from the anaesthetic.
3 Lowered central venous pressure indicates changes in blood volume.

Vomiting and regurgitation

These are problems that can occur postoperatively if the stomach has not been emptied before the operation. Lateral positioning with the head lowered and clearing the nasopharynx by suction will prevent the inhalation of gastric contents.

Restlessness

Restlessness may be an indication of:

1 Anxiety and a need for gentle reassurance.
2 Haemorrhage from the wound.
3 Pain and discomfort from restrictive and tight bandages, creased bedlinen or pressure on the wound.
4 Hypoxia and carbon dioxide retention caused by inadequate respiration.

Postoperative pain

Pain can be relieved by:

1   Adjusting and securing the dressings.
2   Reassurance and constant attention.
3   Warmth and comfort.
4   Administration of prescribed pain relief medication.

Cardiac and respiratory arrest

Irreversible brain damage occurs after three minutes of anoxia. It is therefore important to note the exact time of the arrest.

Signs of cardiopulmonary arrest:

1   Respiratory arrest.
2   Pallor.
3   Absence of a carotid pulse.
4   Fixed and dilated pupils.
5   Unconsciousness in a previously conscious patient.

Procedure in cardiopulmonary arrest

Mouth to mouth breathing to try to re-establish respirations.

1   Call for help and summon the cardiac arrest team.
2   Place the patient on his back with head extended.
3   Pull the patient's jaw forward, establish a clear airway and commence mouth to mouth breathing at the rate of 10–20 exhalations per minute.
4   As soon as possible, continue ventilation with a face mask and Ambu resuscitation bag.

External cardiac massage

Cardiac massage is carried out alternately with mouth to mouth breathing.

1   Strike the sternum once to try to re-establish cardiac function.
2   Place the palm of one hand over the tip of the sternum and the heel of the other hand on top and compress the chest wall.
3   Apply pressure sharply, at the rate of approximately 60 times per minute.
4   Inflate the lungs by mouth to mouth breathing after five compressions of the chest.

5 Continue emergency measures until help arrives or signs of improvement are observed.

The fingers of one hand are sufficient to compress the sternum of a child.

During this procedure the fully equipped mobile resuscitation trolley is brought to the bedside, with the following equipment:

1 Intubation. Endotracheal tubes and connections, airways, face masks, throat spray and magill forceps.
2 Suction catheters.
3 Hypodermic needles, syringes and cannulae of assorted sizes and solutions for intravenous infusion. Sodium bicarbonate and calcium carbonate are available prepackaged, in jet syringes, ready for immediate use.
4 Electrocardiogram electrodes and contact gel.
5 The defibrillator machine and external electrodes.

When the medical team arrives the nurse assists them in their efforts to resuscitate the patient.

The resuscitation equipment is replenished according to the instructions given in the hospital policy for the procedure to follow in a cardiac arrest.

Safety in the recovery room

1 The patient must never be left unattended.
2 Patient trolleys and beds should have a tipping mechanism, restraining rails and locking wheels.
3 All equipment must be tested before use and regularly maintained.
4 All members of the recovery room staff should know the location of the firefighting appliances and resuscitation equipment.
5 The procedure for the care of patients in the event of a fire or explosion should be demonstrated to all the recovery room staff.
6 Fire sheets, or cords, should be placed under the mattresses ready to secure the patient for speedy evacuation in the event of a fire.
7 Incidents and accidents must be reported and recorded.

The transfer of the patient to the ward

When the recorded vital signs indicate that the patient's condition is stable and he is quietly relaxed, arrangements are made for his return to the ward. The recovery nurse makes a verbal report on his present condition and delivers written notes and records to the ward nurse.

A final visit two or three days later, allows the nurse to evaluate the nursing care that she has given in the recovery area and to learn from the patient and from the nursing staff how he has responded to surgery.

Further reading:

Campbell, D and Spence, A (1979) A Nurse's Guide to Anaesthetics, Resuscitation and Intensive Care, 5th edition, Churchill Livingstone

Drain, C B and Shipley, S (1979) The Recovery Room, W B Saunders

CHAPTER 16

MANAGEMENT OF AN OPERATING THEATRE

Objectives

The nurse will be able to:

1 List the factors to be considered in the daily organisation of theatre work.
2 Plan a system for the ordering and storage of sterilised supplies.
3 Adopt a systematic approach to solving problems.
4 Discuss the importance of a planned teaching programme.

Management in the operating theatre

The successful management of an operating theatre is a complex task that demands skills in interpersonal relationships, problem solving and decision making, as well as a thorough knowledge of theatre technology. Whenever a plan of action is contemplated the needs of the patient and of the surgeon have to be considered, in conjunction with the resources available. A number of people are involved and the aim is to create a situation in which each person can perform the job to the best of his or her ability.

Staff in the operating theatre

Orientation

The introduction and welcome that is accorded to anyone entering the operating theatre is more than a courtesy, it is an important responsibility of the theatre staff. The necessity for changing into theatre clothing has to be explained to visitors coming to the theatre for the first time and the areas of the theatre where observers can move without fear of contaminating sterile surfaces has to be clearly defined.

On arrival in the department, new members of staff embark on a planned programme of orientation to acquaint them with the layout and the policies of the department. When these preliminaries have been completed, the theatre sister welcomes the nurse to the operating theatre and introduces her to everyone present so that she is identified and recognised as a member of the team.

Learners in the operating theatre

Written objectives indicate to the learner the skills and knowledge that she can acquire during the period of allocation to the theatre. Plans are made for theoretical teaching, practical experience and methods of assessment, for each learner. The uncertainties of operating theatre schedules and timetables present a real challenge to theatre staff in providing the optimum experience and favourable conditions for learning, but when there are clinical teachers appointed to the theatre they are able to give guidance and valuable assistance with teaching and the arrangement of assignments.

Daily meetings with staff

The leader needs to meet daily with the other members of the team. Everyone can be made fully aware of the part that they will play in the work schedule during a brief meeting held at the start of the day, before operating begins.

Subjects for discussion

1   The allocation of tasks and the responsibilities of each member of the team.
2   The individual needs and problems of each patient.
3   The surgical procedures for the listed operations.

Personal interviews

It is not always easy to find a quiet place for uninterrupted talks during the busy operating day, but opportunities have to be created for talking to individual members of the staff to discuss performance appraisals, assessments and proposals for staff development.

The daily organisation of work

There are so many factors to consider in the daily allocation of jobs that only a planned strategical approach is likely to succeed in providing safety for the patient, efficient assistance for the surgeon and job satisfaction for the staff.

Factors for consideration

1 Assessment of the patient's problems and needs.
2 The appointment of the most suitable person available, to be responsible for each job.
3 The provision of opportunities for learners to gain experience and to practise skills.
4 Arrangements for the supervision and support of learners.
5 Consideration for the problems of the surgeons. Junior doctors and surgeons who are fatigued at the end of the day need the assistance of an experienced scrub nurse.
6 The provision of variety and opportunities for fresh experiences to motivate staff and stimulate interest.
7 Arrangements for the staff to take regular breaks for refreshment and relaxation.

Organisation

Careful planning and logical thinking are the key to good organisation. Every activity has to be considered so that it can be accomplished with an economy of movement and yet maintain the high standards that are obligatory for the delivery of patient care that is as efficient at the end of the session as at the beginning.

Simple and uncomplicated schemes have the best chance of success provided that information is conveyed clearly and assurances are given that the directions have been received and understood.

Storage of supplies

Systems in which items are grouped together in types and arranged according to the frequency of their use, will prevent repeated to and fro movements that are a real hazard to the maintenance of asepsis in the theatre.

Ordering and controlling stock

The management of the stock supplied to the theatre entails close cooperation with personnel in the supplies departments of the hospital. Policies are devised to establish routine collection and delivery services and the methods to be used for submitting orders. These mutually agreed arrangements must be adhered to by everyone using the services, if the schemes are to operate successfully. Many of the items, such as linen and sterilised bowls, are recycled and returned for further use and interruption of this cycle, by stockpiling, can jeopardise the system and prove to be very costly.

Guidelines in stock control

1   Plan comprehensive, simple and easy-to-follow systems.
2   Accurately record the quantities ordered and those received.
3   Check stock and complete orders regularly at a prearranged time of day, or day of the week.
4   Despatch recycled articles as soon as possible after use.
5   Review stock usage regularly and adjust stock levels when necessary.
6   Maintain adequate stocks only and return surplus supplies.

Planning a system for ordering from a sterilising department

1   Plan the arrangement of stock in suitable storage spaces.
2   Determine the length of time that will elapse between deliveries (e.g. 24 hours).
3   Estimate appropriate stock levels by calculating the number of each item required during the period of time between deliveries.
4   Label the shelf or container for each item with the stock level number.
5   Compose a list of all the items supplied by the sterilising department.
6   Set a time for the daily counting of stock remaining on the shelves and completing the order form.
7   Retain a copy of the order.
8   Check the supplies delivered against the number ordered.

Recording information

A great deal of information can be stored on small cards that are easily filed and readily accessible (Figure 16.1).

Subjects can be grouped in types and alphabetically arranged, to

SCREWS Bone   Type.... Sherman

Description   Catalogue No.....

Titanium

Length 34 mm
Diameter 4 mm

Manufacturer................. Address.................

Stock Record Card

Quantity	Date Ordered	Date Delivered	Remarks
20	8.10.80	15.12.80	delivery delayed
30	17.1.81.	20.2.81.	....

Reverse Side of Record Card

Figure 16.1 Stock record card.

present a system that is simple to operate and will provide a reliable reference that is essential for estimation of the cost of procedures and in budgeting for future expenditure.

1 List the information that is required.
2 Plan the layout of the card.
3 Use a separate card for each item.
4 Record accurately and precisely.
5 Fix markers to the cards to denote problems or queries.
6 Use colour coding for groups of similar articles.

Problem solving

Knowledge and experience are valuable assets in the solving of problems and making decisions but unless the problems are approached systematically, the results can bring confusion and dissatisfaction. An intellectual approach similar to that used in the nursing process can be applied to management.

A systematic approach to problems

1 Aim. Clearly define, in writing, the problem and the aim.
2 Enquire. Collect all the information on the subject that is available.
3 Specify. State exactly what you need to know.
4 Plan. Write plans indicating who will perform the action and at what time and place.
5 Act. Implement the plan as soon as possible.
6 Review. Examine the results to ascertain whether the aims were achieved.

Decisions

Apparently complex problems can be simplified by systematically analysing the situation to establish the ultimate goal. Alternative, possible, courses of action can then be considered and a decision made by selecting the most appropriate option.

Aids to effective management

1 Keep accurate accounts.
2 Plan and work methodically.
3 Communicate effectively.
4 Seek information on new developments.
5 Participate in the activities of the unit, the hospital, and national nursing associations.
6 Review results constantly.

Essential qualities for success in management

1 Empathy and consideration for other people.
2 Integrity and honesty.
3 Confidence and an ability to motivate others.
4 Perseverance to achieve objectives.
5 Flexibility and preparedness to accept change when it is necessary.

Teaching in the operating theatre

Theatre sisters and qualified staff in the theatres have a commitment to participate in the teaching and training of staff in the department. Although basic facts and principles can be taught in the classroom, the specialised skills and techniques can only be learnt by practical experience in the clinical setting of the operating theatre during surgery. It is here that the true concept of asepsis is experienced and nurses can fully appreciate the responsibility of caring for unconscious patients.

By establishing clearly-expressed objectives the teaching can be controlled and planned to meet the individual needs of the learner.

Example
Objective: After completing two weeks' allocation to the theatre the nurse will be able to correctly open sterile packs.

Qualified members of the staff should acquire skills in teaching so that the unique knowledge possessed by them is conveyed to the learner by the most effective means, and allocation to the operating theatre is a rewarding and beneficial experience.

The learning environment
The atmosphere and tempo of a busy operating theatre is confusing to a newcomer but a carefully planned programme of introduction and orientation that includes instruction in the wearing of theatre clothing and a tour of the rooms and the facilities of the department, will reassure the apprehensive learner.

Preliminary teaching on the basic principles of infection control and safety precautions in the theatres can most effectively be taught in the classroom, with the aid of illustrations from books and audiovisual apparatus.

Demonstration of skills
All the members of the theatre team should be able to demonstrate a skill to someone who is unfamiliar with the procedure or the equipment.

1 State exactly what you are aiming to do.
2 Plan the demonstration and collect the equipment.
3 Prepare everything in a logical order.
4 Explain the principles and reasons for the actions.
5 Demonstrate each component of the equipment.

6 Demonstrate each stage separately and confirm that it has been understood.
7 Allow the learner to imitate each stage before proceeding to the next.
8 Repeat the entire procedure.
9 Allow the learner to practise the procedure without interruption.
10 Evaluate the performance.
11 Prepare for further practice, if it is required.

Guidelines for successful instruction

1 Allow sufficient time for the instruction.
2 Use simple basic terms.
3 Be realistic and do not attempt to include more information than can be assimilated by the learner in the time available.
4 Whenever possible stand beside the learner, facing in the same direction.
5 Give praise, where due, and encouragement, when assessing the learner's performance.

Assessment

Assessing the progress of learners is an integral part of the teaching programme requiring time and forethought if the assessment is to be valid and helpful to the teacher and the learner.

A planned assessment

A test or an assessment that is nervously anticipated, does not reveal a true measure of the learner's ability to perform in the practical situation, but it is sometimes necessary to make arrangements in advance for an assessment to take place at a particular time that is convenient to the assessor and will not disrupt the organisation of the theatre.

Continuous assessment

Continuous assessment monitors and records the learners progress at every stage and indicates when changes in teaching methods or extra practice are needed, if the objectives are to be achieved. The practical skills and the attitude of the learner can be observed and fairly assessed when the tasks are performed in the clinical situation.

Assessment of learner's performance	Learner score	Teacher score
1. Accurately tested the diathermy and suction apparatus		
2. Maintained asepsis when opening sterile packs		
3. Correctly assessed the physical needs of the patient		
4. Provided the necessary supports for positioning		
5. Participated in swab and instrument counts according to hospital procedure		
6. Promptly supplied the scrub nurses needs		
Please rate the performance on a scale of 1 to 5 and note comments on the reverse side of this sheet 5 = excellent 4 = good, satisfactory standard 3 = requires more care 2 = below required standard 1 = unsatisfactory		

Figure 16.2   Example of learner's self-assessment form.

Self-assessment

Theatre nurses have to use their own judgement and be discerning when they are making decisions, and self-assessment develops these qualities.

The learner is asked to recall the procedure and grade her performance on a prearranged scale (Figure 16.2) or to make a verbal assessment and suggest ways in which she would aim to improve if the procedure was repeated.

The discussion that is initiated by this assessment is a valuable guide to the effectiveness of the teaching and encourages articulate communication and logical thinking by the learner.

Peer assessment

Assessment of the standards of work and the attitudes of one's peers is a difficult and precarious activity requiring courage, and experience in the art of assessing, but it is a method currently being advocated to encourage qualified staff to maintain high standards, and in auditing the quality of patient care in the operating theatre.

The assessment of a skill

1 Consider each stage of the procedure under a separate heading and record a score or make written notes.
2 Observe closely and continuously.
3 Allow the learner to complete the task without interruptions.
4 Discuss the assessment with the learner and give her an opportunity to state the reasons for her actions.
5 Adjust the teaching programme if necessary.

Further reading

Drucker, P F (1968) The Practice of Management, Pan
Russell, G J (1972) Teaching in Further Education, Pitman

CHAPTER 17

RESEARCH IN NURSING

Objectives

The nurse will be able to:

1 List the stages in the basic research method.
2 Identify the methods used for data collection in research reports.
3 Describe the practical aspects to be considered in writing a report of a research study.
4 Enumerate the pitfalls and the ethical problems that may be encountered by the researcher.

Research in nursing

Research is a relatively new and exciting aspect of nursing that has been encouraged and developed since the 1960s. It involves a systematic search for information that can be utilised in education and in the formation of policies and procedures. Practising and following the research method increases the nurse's ability to analyse critically and to make judgements that are substantiated by facts. These are skills that are required by all theatre nurses and are particularly valuable in auditing the quality of care in the operating theatre.

Fulltime research teams, with financial support and technical resources have conducted large-scale research in nursing, and smaller studies, made by practising nurses, have also contributed to our nursing knowledge. Some operating theatre nurses have grasped the opportunities that are offered, through scholarships and awards, to complete studies that have led to the development of plans for the improvement of patient care, but there are some activities in operating theatre nursing that are perpetuated by habit and have never been studied to establish that they are effective or necessary.

Nurses have an obligation to study and evaluate research reports that are relevant to their speciality but this can only be satisfactorily achieved by acquiring some knowledge of the basic research method and the skills involved.

The basic research method

The eight stages of the research method represent a sequential and logical approach to the subject.

Definition of the problem

This is a task that can be difficult and exacting, but one that must be completed satisfactorily before proceeding to the next stage. Although a broad statement of the problem may seem to be acceptable for the title this will need to be further defined and expressed in detail, to avoid confusion in the later stages when there is a considerable amount of data to be analysed.

Survey of the literature

The systematic search begins by making a survey of the relevant literature, and contacting people with specialised knowledge of the subject. Text books often include a section on history and development, and extracts from journals reveal current opinions and lead to reports on recent research. Manufacturers of medical products are helpful in supplying technical data and information on the production and trials of new products.

Every piece of information must be recorded at the time of discovery with details of the source, the author and the date of publication.

The planning

This is the stage when decisions have to be made and plans are completed in detail.

1 The selection of the type of investigation that will be most appropriate for the subject.
2 The defining of objectives or the formulating of an hypothesis.

3 The compiling of a timetable with proposed dates for the completion of each stage and the date by which it is estimated that the final report will be ready.

4 Selection of the methods that will be employed for the collection of data.

5 An estimation of the financial cost of the project.

The pilot study

Whenever it is possible the proposed plans are tested by conducting a mini-research project, following the stages of the research method, to produce a small sample of the study that is contemplated.

The results of the pilot study may reveal problems in organisation or difficulties in data collection that can be rectified before the main project is launched.

The collection of data

There are various methods of collecting information, one or more of which may be used in each research study.

Observation The researcher records the activities of a particular group of people while she acts as an observer or participates in the action.

Consultation Previous work on the subject is investigated by consulting books, pictures and existing records.

Interviews A planned set of verbal questions that will be put to participants can be prepared before the interview. The replies to these straightforward questions can be easily summarised so that comparisons can be made.

Unstructured interviews evoke the most spontaneous response, when the answers to questions are invited during free conversation, but the distractions and omissions that can occur may result in variations that are difficult to record and summarise.

Questionnaires Questionnaires that require written replies can be widely distributed, but the form must be carefully prepared and tested by a pilot study, to ensure that the directions clearly state what is required of the participants and that the questions are not ambiguous or liable to be misinterpreted.

Questionnaires are designed to include:

1   A brief statement of introduction explaining the nature and the aims of the study.
2   An assurance that all information will be treated confidentially.
3   A guarantee that the respondent can remain anonymous.
4   Space provided for the comments of participants.
5   An expression of gratitude for help and cooperation received.

The ethics of research

Researchers have an obligation to respect the rights of people to consent, or to refuse, to participate in the research or to withdraw their consent at any point in the study. Consideration must be given to the possibility that questioning could, in some circumstances, cause mental stress or that investigation could be regarded as an invasion of privacy.

Analysing the data

The collected data has to be sorted and grouped to present a visual record of the information. Tables and charts, as well as statistical symbols, are used to clarify and explain variations and to show comparisons. The analysing process is a time consuming activity that can be rendered more accurate and accomplished more quickly by the use of data recording equipment and computers.

The conclusion

The researcher draws conclusions from the evidence that is presented by the analysis of the data. Proposals for change may be indicated or recommendations for further research using different methods. The work is evaluated to ascertain whether the objectives were achieved and the hypothesis was proved to be correct.

Writing the report

The report is written under the same headings, and in the same order as the stages of the research method with the following additions:

1   A page bearing the title of the study and the names of the author and coresearchers.
2   A list of the contents.
3   An introduction to the report.

4   Copies of questionnaires and a list of the specific questions asked at interviews.
5   A bibliography and details of references.

Pitfalls in practising the research method

1   Failure to complete stage one and define the subject in detail before proceeding.
2   Omitting to conduct a pilot study.
3   Failure to plan realistically or in sufficient detail.
4   Underestimating the time required to summarise and analyse the data.
5   Failure to allow sufficient time for writing the report.
6   Making the study too 'wide' and embracing aspects that are not directly related to the project.

Nurses who read and evaluate research reports are continually adding to their knowledge and are well qualified to participate in assessing the value and effectiveness of procedures and products.

Research is a highly specialised subject that invites and deserves further study through the excellent books and papers that have been published and it is hoped that theatre nurses will have the opportunity to actively participate in research studies, or perhaps to conduct some research of their own. There is great satisfaction and a sense of achievement in being so closely involved in a search for new knowledge that can be utilised for the improvement of patient care.

Further reading

Clark, J and Hockey, L (1980) Research for Nursing, HM&M
Guidelines to Research in Nursing, Numbers 1 to 6, King Edwards Hospital Fund for London
Joint Board of Clinical Nursing Studies, the Research Objective in Joint Board Courses
Royal College of Nursing, Research publications, The Royal College of Nursing of the United Kingdom

INDEX